CU00703888

AWAKENING THE TRANQUIL WARRIOR

APPLYING ANCESTRAL NUTRITION, QUANTUM BIOLOGY, MEDITATION, AND MINDFUL FITNESS TO UNLOCK YOUR FULL POTENTIAL

Trenton Sweet

&

Kaitlyn Sweet

Awakening the Tranquil Warrior

Copyright © 2022 by Trenton Sweet and Kaitlyn Sweet

All rights reserved. No part of this book may be reproduced or transmitted in any form or by any means without written permission from the authors.

ISBN# 978-1-0880-6160-2

Dedications

Maelyn, you are our first born, you are the reason this book was written. When your mom and I found out you were on your way it changed our lives in ways that we never expected. You are a true blessing, and we love you with everything that we are. You are a powerful light, and we will help you shine bright your whole life, no matter what you need. You are a young child at the time of this writing, and you have taught us more than any teacher we have ever had. You are an intuitive and intellectual warrior and it's easy to see that your instinct and understanding will lead you through an amazing life. We can't wait to see who you become. Your spirit animals are a unicorn and a mermaid, this is what you tell us. You have the love, compassion, and joy that I would expect these creatures to express so I believe it to be true.

Wade, my only boy. You wild son of a gun! You carry the Sweet surname on your shoulders, don't let that weigh on you though because you've got a thousand ancestors guiding you each step of the way. You are a true lion, strong headed, proud, and full of passion. You are just like your Grandpa Sweet's son whether you like it or not. In doing my best to teach you to be a man, you have taught me what it truly means to be one. Your love and compassion will have you leading with your heart, and we can't wait to see who you will become, at this writing you are also a young child. We love you with everything that we are. I know that your heart will guide you to places both beautiful and difficult, whatever you need, we will be there. Your spirit animals are a lion and a dragon, this is what you tell us. You have the heart, strength, and fire of both creatures, so we believe it to be true.

Rosalia, you are the baby, the youngest of the Sweet's. You have an amazing spirit that drives us to be better every day. Your eyes are so clearly loving and connected; the galaxy is within them. Your baby smile and giggles bring pure joy to our souls. You are 4 months old at the time of this writing and it is obvious that your spiritual divinity is powerful. Your spiritual intuitiveness will lead you through an incredible life. We can't wait to see who you become. We love you with everything that we are. We will be there for you no matter what you need. A spiritual friend of your moms told her that your spirit animal is an eagle. You already display the wisdom, pride, and respect that an eagle represents, let that spirit guide you and fly high and proud forever little one.

TABLE OF CONTENTS

PREFACE

Have you ever picked up a book that promises to turn you into the "baddest mother fucker alive"? Like this book says that Kaitlyn and I will awaken the Tranquil Warrior that you wish to be. You start reading it and throughout the whole book it just tells you over and over again that they will tell you how and what to do in a later chapter, but that later chapter never comes? Me too. They start out claiming that they can change your life in millions of powerful ways all you've got to do is keep reading. This is obnoxious as hell. So, keep on reading and by the end of this book I will tell you how to change your life and awaken your Tranquil Warrior with no bounds.

Just kidding. I'm going to give you and your family the starter pack right here before you dive into the book so that you can start making positive changes in your day-to-day life right now. Some of us are speed readers and some of us are not. Sometimes I can read a book front to back in a day and sometimes a single book can sit on my nightstand for a couple months. Normally, when I pick up a book there's a reason why. If I'm picking up a book titled *Awakening the Tranquil Warrior* that's probably what I want to become and I want to become that warrior sooner than later.

I'll give you what you can do today to start awakening the Tranquil Warrior that lives within you. And throughout the rest of the book, I will tell you why I believe taking these simple steps will elevate your entire being.

Warrior: A person engaged or experienced in warfare. Essentially, a person who fights in battles and is known for having courage and skill. (Merriam-Webster) So what does it mean to be a "Tranquil Warrior"? For beginners, we are ALL warriors. Every one of us is engaged in and has been engaged in many battles throughout our lives, some of which we have won without a doubt, others were epic losses, and some battles we fight our entire lives. Secondly, in a way believe it or not you are courageous and skillful in the art of war. Each battle you've won, day in and day out you do so skillfully and courageously. The warrior part is established in each of us, now we must awaken and enlighten that warrior.

A Tranquil Warrior has the ability to defeat all potential opponents without fear or fault. Yet stays peaceful in the face of demons. An individual that can control their own emotions in the heat of battle. Staying focused, un-shook, and un-triggered at all times. Presenting their best physical, emotional, and spiritual fitness. Tranquil literally means "Free from disturbances; calm." To be a tranquil warrior you must do the following.

- Limit your *processed sugar* intake right now. If you can cut *processed* sugar from your diet all together then do so. Limiting your processed sugar intake will not only decrease inflammation in your body but will increase the OVERALL function of your body. This doesn't mean replacing those processed sugars with fake ones with *zero calories*, they can be just as bad if not worse for you, and they are still "processed". Fresh fruits are good sugars, "table sugars" are bad sugars. Sugar is addictive and very destructive so limit and then eliminate its consumption. Do it now. More on this in a later chapter.

- Increase your time in the sun with fewer clothes and no sunglasses. If you have sensitive skin, then you can start with the early morning and evening sunshine. Increase time in the sun as your body adapts. Properly hydrating with minerals and fresh whole foods/including animal foods will help a lot with your sensitivity to the sun. Try sun gazing with your eyes closed staring directly at the sun. Try 1-to-5-minute intervals to start with. Without the sun there would be no life; without the sun *you* would have no life. Utilize the glorious sun to improve your life and do not use generic sunscreens. If you can eat meals outdoors in the sun do so starting now. If you can take a leisurely walk in the sun after a meal incorporate that as well. This is a good time to squeeze in those pesky phone calls that would otherwise be made indoors.

- Get grounded. Everyday spend time in direct contact with mother earth. You can achieve this through being barefoot or sitting on the ground or even wearing shoes that are conductive to the earth's energy like leather. Preferably not rubber or synthetics. Swimming in a natural source of water like a river, lake, or ocean is even better. If you can mix sun gazing or "tanning" with your grounding practice you can double up on time efficacy and positive changes. If you're really pressed for time another way that you can elevate your grounding game is to purchase a grounding sheet or a grounding mat to place on your bed or in your workspace or even in your vehicle that you can sit on, that you plug in directly to your outlet into the grounding source, this simulates the same effect of actually grounding and can increase the amount of time you spend grounded daily to help with inflammation, anxiety, depression and more.

- Move your body. The human organism is designed to move in a multitude of complex ways in quick powerful bouts as well as endurance bouts. The human body functions more efficiently when it is moved in such ways. Make it a part of your daily routine to move in ways that your regular life does not incorporate. Such as, lunging, twisting, jumping, throwing, squatting, swinging, hinging, pressing, pulling, sprinting etc. Moving your body in strange and different ways every day will help basically every other system in your body to function more efficiently. making you as a whole function more efficiently.

- Breathe. Don't forget this one or you might suffocate. Really though. Breathing exercises are one of my favorite ways to improve respiratory function and fitness. Breathwork also alleviates stress, anxiety, depression, and more mental ailments. I love breathwork because no matter your fitness level, you can still breath. Or else you'd be, well dead. Do the following practice at your own pace, if you feel as though you may pass out then start at lighter increments. Take a good 20-40 breaths at three to four second inhale lengths, to an immediate exhale breath of proportion to your inhale and then on your chosen final exhale hold your breath for as long as you can (work on increasing this time as your practice continues) then take a long FULL inhale and hold that breath for 10-20 seconds. Then start again. If you are aware of the Ice Man Wim Hof then you will recognize this routine as he is the cultivator of it. Another one of my favorite breathwork practices is box breathing (4 seconds inhale, 4 seconds hold, 4 seconds exhale, 4 seconds hold & repeat) a few times a day or for several minutes at a time. You don't have to make a perfect breathing regimen just be mindful about your breathing. DO NOT MOUTH BREATHE. If you are a mouth breather stop doing that right now. You should breathe through your nose almost exclusively, filling up your belly (lower chest and diaphragm) and you should be breathing at a consistent but calm rate.

- Limit your screen time. If your job entails staring into a LED, blue light toxic screen for hours on end I suggest you buy a blue light blocking screen protector and a pair of blue light blocking glasses. Every 30 minutes or so (set a timer if necessary) look off into the distance at something 20ft or so away and focus on it for 30 seconds, just to give your eyes a rest. Take a moment to close your eyes and lightly press on them with your palms. Take a day, a week, or every couple of weeks and unplug entirely when possible. The modern world has screens everywhere so this one is tricky, but just limiting your average screen time down a couple hours a week will make a big difference. This especially goes for your kiddos. This should go without saying, but when we are limiting screen time the most beneficial time to let go of is the media time. No matter what tribalistic side you place yourself on, you are being targeted and fear mongered by news media outlets. The constant stress associated with this is deteriorating your health.

- Cut vegetable oil, palm oil, canola/rapeseed oil, soybean oil consumption. If you have anything labeled vegetable oil, canola oil, soybean oil or palm oil in your cabinet toss that sucker in the trash. This is tough when it comes to boxed and processed foods so start with what you cook with. Don't cook with those anymore. Stop it. Go buy some fruit oils like olive, or coconut oil. I personally love animal fats like tallow, lard, butter, ghee, or suet. Choose labels like organic, pasture raised, grass-fed and finished, and local when possible.

- Choose organic. Organic means, minimal or no pesticides, non-GMO, no growth hormones, antibiotics or artificial fertilizers, Pesticides are a slow human killer. They *kill* pests. Pests that are

13

akin to humans in many ways, pesticides in small amounts won't kill you right away but they will slowly damage you and your DNA. Many fertilizers and pesticides that we consume don't just hurt us and then get flushed out immediately, many ingredients stay in the body and continue to damage us for years. Even rinsing non-organic foods doesn't get rid of all the pesticides, they soak into the plant through its skin, its roots suck them inside of them. If its GMO, pesticides can literally be a part of the plant's genetic makeup. Antibiotics don't just disappear from products either, we consume them, and they impact our bodies in the same way they impacted the animal's body.

- Eat more like your ancestors. YOUR ancestors. If you have a general idea of what hemisphere of the world the bulk of your ancestors came from, then eat like them. Not like the ones within the last five thousand years. More like the ancestor's pre-agriculture. In fact, try to live in a relative manner to them, without giving up todays' luxuries of course. Learn about them and the way in which they lived. Get rid of toxic cookware like Teflon coated pots and pans. Choose cast iron. Choose glass over plastic whenever possible. Drink your water at room temperature, not plain either, as the Author of "Minimize Injury, Maximize Performance, a sports parents survival guide" Tommy John III says, "Not plain fucking water". Adding something as simple as sea salt, lemon/lime juice to your water will amplify your hydration. Teas, smoothies, or just plain fresh fruit soaking in your water. Note that a large bulk of your hydration should be coming from your food. (We love using trace mineral drops to increase quality hydration in our home.)

- Don't over sanitize. Your immune system depends on it. Cut the use of soaps and cleaning products of ALL KINDS in your household that contain

14

fluoride, aluminum, parabens, sulfates, phthalates, formaldehyde, phenoxyethanol, alcohols and polyethylene glycol. Soaps you are using on your body should be edible (I ate Irish Spring as a kid for being bad, I lived, but it is not technically edible). Seriously though, your body soap should be edible. They should be basic, oils like olive, avocado, coconut, MCT, tallow, lard, ghee, cacao butter, etc. Maybe a soft exfoliator like charcoal or salt, water, and pot ash or something similar. No sugar as an exfoliator. Your household cleaning products should be very similar to your hygiene products although many household chores require something more powerful, I suggest using items that contain vinegars or naturally occurring acids like those found in lemons. Dental hygiene products are the same. Your skin is the largest organ in the human body, it soaks in its entire environment especially what is lathered on to it with open pores from a hot shower or hot sun. Your skins micro-biome is arguably the most important part of your immune system, don't kill it with sanitizers and cleaning products.

- This final bullet is for the family man or woman, or even grandma or grandpa, or guardian in general over more than just yourself a significant other and maybe an animal. lead by example, if you want to be healthy and you want your family to be healthy then you must practice what you preach all the time when eyes are on you and when eyes are off you. I highly recommend that if you are married or live with a significant other that you start this journey together as it can be difficult at mealtime to eat, say, a swordfish filet with a fresh tomato grown locally, while your significant other is eating a stuffed waffle covered in syrup and whipped cream. this also means that you must go all in. it's like taking an ice plunge you can't just dip your toes in and expect to comfortably sink the rest of your body in over time. This is something that you must dive into. To start I recommend going through your cabinets and throwing away anything that you have with vegetable oils in them. Especially if you're currently cooking with any of those. Go to your cabinets and any food items you have that contain more than 5 grams of added sugar per serving throw away. Learn how to cook with fruit oils and animal fats. Make this an experience for your family and your children. As we know, when we incorporate the whole family into a task, children can learn, have fun, and grow from these types of experiences. This will help get the rest of the family on board with this new style of living and especially this new style of eating. Exercise with your spouse and your children whenever possible, especially your kids, let them see you being active and having FUN doing it. This will encourage them to do the same. If you have your kids in sports or they're in school don't rely on those sports or gym class to get them their daily exercise, because a lot of that time is spent learning rather than exercising. Make your life active and then include actual physical exercise. When you're at the grocery store allow your children to pick out items that they like, if something doesn't fit your new restrictions and guidelines then find something similar that does and help them to find substitutions for the foods that they enjoy. Just like you are finding substitutions for the foods that you enjoy. This doesn't have to be hard, in fact it should be fun. As far as outdoor activities go our children love obstacle courses and scavenger hunts. Plan adventure days and let your children help you do so. Get the whole family in the sunshine, barefoot and smiling.

This should get you started down the Tranquil Warrior path. If you have been blessed with children take a moment to consider the current health epidemics facing our youth. Obesity, mental health disorders, and issues stemming from them are intensifying with each generation. This is caused and exasperated by lack of direct sunlight, not moving like we were designed, limited contact with nature, and ancestrally inconsistent diets. An excess of processed sugars, stress, blue flickering artificial light, and EMFs.

What we do throughout our lives will be passed on to our offspring, all the damage, all the trauma, and most importantly for our journey, all the positive adaptations as well. It is utterly important for you to change yourself first, but it is also important to help our suffering youth regain their tranquil warrior ability. It starts with you and spreads out to everyone you spend time around. Use the steps above to dramatically increase your entire family's health today.

INTRODUCTION

I grew up primarily in a small town in Northern Michigan with two working parents. My mother worked in and around the school system, so I saw her quite a bit. She drove my brother and I around since her hours were similar to our school hours. She was (and is) sweet, empathetic, supportive, caring, and helpful. Her empathetic sovereignty meant that my brother and I would get drug around taking care of the elders in our family as they were nearing death, doing extra chores for family members. Her compassion is one of her best attributes. I learned a lot from these experiences taking care of the elders in their dying days. Though these lessons would be misplaced until I grew up, I learned the value of life and time.

Despite eating some meals from the local food pantry and wearing clothes from consignment stores my mom always seemed to keep it together, at least in front of us kids. My father's job and parenting style was the perfect opposition to hers. He worked in an iron factory, working longer and harder hours than most and would often pick up what overtime he could. He would come home in an all-blue uniform, covered in iron dust and soot. I literally thought he was Ironman, and he never argued that he wasn't. He despised that we would get some supplemental food from the local pantries and clothes from consignment shops. He worked so hard for what we had. As little as it may have been, there was a significant amount of pride in it. He loved(s) to tell stories of our ancestry, both recent and archaic. He always tried to be around, though the work and stress could make him somewhat testy. One thing that always sparked his attention was when we would defend someone less fortunate, win a fight, or do well in a sporting event. He would tell stories of his childhood, and his fathers' life where they had carried out similar feats. My brothers and I would be sitting there, eyes glazed over, hanging on to every word. My dad has always been a great storyteller.

He loved it and we did too, there is something natural, special, and beneficial for a young man having a masculine figure to look up to. Mine was always my father. As I try now to teach my children not to let anyone push them around or manipulate them, I find myself rewarding the same types of behavior. Those vigilante or hero like behaviors. This was a double-edged sword for me growing up, I started to seek out these situations where I could reap the rewards of heroism. I would fight with anyone growing up, middle-aged men at the basketball court, teachers, kids from out of town etc. anyone that I thought was treating me or someone else unfairly was fair game.

Over the years this became a part of who I was, chasing that next dopamine rush or reward. Internally I craved that feeling. Unconsciously of course. If there wasn't a "bad guy" around and I wasn't competing in a sport I would find a bad guy or fight with myself. If you understand the law of attraction, then you know that what you seek is what you find. It turned into an addiction to adrenaline, but in an anger driven way, at least the energy and emotional drive that goes with it.

The fighting wasn't my only adrenaline outlet. I started to excel in athletics where I could basically fight without the repercussions and would even earn accolades for intense aggression. During this time, I found that through extreme physical exhaustion I could get a sort of runners high, or high in general. This led me to excruciatingly long runs in the dead of winter where I vividly remember passing out at the top of a hill in a snowbank after vomiting because I pushed my body too far, I was doing air squats at every stop sign and pushups in the snow every time a car passed. As odd as it sounds, I found great pleasure in the exhaustion. My mind would slip into this meditative, euphoric, "flow" like state where nothing else mattered except for me and the task at hand. I could zero in on any goal like an eagle on a rabbit. Sometimes it got out of hand I'll admit but I did enjoy it.

I almost drowned myself in Lake Bellaire one fall around the age of 15. I had dreams of being an elite athlete and I had heard, read, and seen on TV that the best athletes pushed themselves incredibly hard to achieve greatness. With that motivation and the developing addiction to adrenaline, I took off on my bike about 3 miles from our house to the lake. I parked my bike at the park and ran about 5 miles around town and back (for roughly 45 minutes), grabbed the monkey bars and went back and forth between pullups and pushups until I could barely move my arms, got back on the trail, and ran as fast as I could, as far as I could. Then jogged back. When I got back to the park my chest and back were still heavy and tired, but I didn't care, I grabbed the monkey bars and went for another round of pullups and pushups. My testosterone and adrenaline driven brain suggested I dive into the lake and swim across and back as a final test to my athleticism before riding my bike home. The swimming buoys suggested I stay in one specific area, but my mind knew no limits. The frigid water took my breath away and in just a few breast strokes I realized I had made a mistake. I got just outside the buoys and my chest cramped up, I flipped over to try a back stroke, since I *had* to complete what I had set out to do. It didn't take many strokes this direction until my back and shoulders also cramped and I was left treading water with very little gas in the tank. I knew at this moment I had pushed it too far, no one else was at the park, no one in the lake, just me, incapable of moving my arms in any efficient manner, treading water desperately trying to get back to shore. My legs began to cramp, and I started to panic. Dropping well below the surface several times on my way to shore. Once I got to shore, I laid there gasping for air and trying frantically to resolve the intense cramping I was now feeling practically everywhere. I don't know how long exactly I laid there but it felt like hours of thinking "how am I going to ride my bike home like this?". I eventually limped beside my bike using it as a wheeled crutch.

The stupid limits I pushed had led me to some decent feats in school. Setting some records for our Friday "long distance runs" and "Strongest man in school" my senior year where we did a legit strong man competition pulling Humvees and flipping tires etc.

The only thing I thought I knew about fitness at that time was that I needed to push my body to excruciating limits to get stronger and faster. I knew almost nothing about nutrition, I ate probably 85% carbs (mostly processed), 10% protein, and 5% fats. My body was starving for real nutrients, and I had no idea. I did have a realization at one point though that all the work I was putting in should have been doing more for me so, I bought a body building book written by Bill Pearl and started doing the workouts he described. Pushing my body to its limits became a habit, only now, I had specific routines.

A passion burned for football during this time, after my senior season I found out that a Minor League football team was moving to the closest city to my hometown. I knew that this was my next chapter. My grades were good enough to stay in sports but bad enough that a college scholarship wasn't in the cards.

My Mom and Dad drove me to tryouts to an indoor facility where we went through an NFL combine type session. At the time I was only 5' 7" and about 170lbs. My adrenaline seeking youth had led me to near hypothermic runs in the dead of winter, extremely long, and dangerous swimming sessions in frigid Northern Michigan waters and grueling sessions in gyms and a general lack of accepting when to stop. I lived the "no pain, no gain" mantra. My training was intense, maybe a little too intense and not exactly sport specific but the intensity and drive was there none the less. I performed well compared to the other athletes.

My father to this day still tells the story about the day of tryouts. Dad - "He was by far the smallest man there, the fastest but for sure the smallest. Youngest too. They did all their skills, running and jumping stuff and I thought, yeah, he did okay in those tests. Then it was time for the weight-lifting part. Trenton walked up to the bench and the spotters there only had one plate on each side for him and he goes, "I want the 225" and the big dudes there both looked at each other and laughed at him, saying something like "yeah, right!?" And he nodded his head and said something that I couldn't hear from where I was, the two guys shrugged their shoulders and loaded up the bar with two more plates, he laid on the bench and knocked out like 25 reps! Everyone spotting and judging that test was amazed and I knew from there that he had made the team." The egotistical part of me always loves hearing him tell this story. I can only imagine the pride I would have for my son looking back at the odds he had faced. I earned myself a spot despite the odds, that I didn't even realize were stacked against me. I was the smallest and the youngest, I was from a poor family in a very small town, I was not the fastest nor the strongest nor the best skilled despite my father's interpretation. Nor do I remember repping 225 pounds 25 times, but I'll take it. Now I was the Semi-Pro athlete wearing a crown at our high school prom with lots of good friends and a bright future ahead of me.

I played for two years as a strong safety and did alright. During this time, I moved to that city about 45 minutes from my hometown, enrolled in a community college and moved into the equivalent of a crack house with a friend. Seriously. It was just as "bad news" as you could imagine. My adrenaline seeking days quickly expanded to include a lot of alcohol and marijuana with an occasional pre-game substance. I was 18-20 during this period and I spent almost all of my time outside of working and football, partying, drinking, smoking, chewing (since freshman year of high school) and fighting. I didn't leave anytime for education. I flunked out before my second semester even started. I was working as a lifeguard at a local water park in the winter and a Golf Course running equipment in the summer and could barely pay rent.

The semi-professional athlete's life is not so glorious, the money is basically non-existent for most and for the team I was on it was literally nonexistent for me. We got paid royalties on products sold with our name on them, but the team was wise to never put anyone's name on any merchandise they sold. They did pay for uniforms, travel expenses like rental cars, bussing and lodging. But besides that, it was on me. I thought that this was the step right before becoming an NFL player, and for some maybe it is. This minor league, I quickly learned was filled with a lot of great athletes that had gotten themselves in legal trouble, bad grades that kept em out of college (like me), badly injured, or even played at the next level but again got themselves hurt, or in a lot of trouble. And ended up in the minor leagues as well as a lot of guys just having fun competing again. The experience shaped who I was becoming and left imprints in my life to guide me through many future tribulations.

My rent was ridiculously cheap at just 90 dollars a month and yet I was having trouble paying it. I was constantly trying to fix up a car from a scrap heap so I could drive to work and practice. Between the malnourishment of poor food choices and the adrenaline seeking destruction my health was declining rapidly. Adrenal fatigue was setting in. Before I was 20!? I didn't know it by that term at the time, but I knew that I had hit a wall. Something had to change, I just didn't know what or why.

My best friend had moved to the Appalachia region to work in the then lucrative oil and gas industry. I hadn't talked to him much for the year or so he had been gone and then one night in late fall he showed up to the "crack house" in a nice, newer f-150 and some sweet new cowboy boots. I was in shock; this was the same dude that used to drive to the even more poor parts of Michigan with me to buy cheap weed to flip for a profit in our hometown. And here he was all cleaned up and driving a nice truck. We got caught up over a few drinks and he told me that he could use a hand down there. The pay was 11 dollars an hour. A three dollar raise from I was. They offered "company housing" and I would be getting well over 100 hours a week. A poor boy from Northern Michigan started seeing money signs. I was thinking about how I could make over 50k a year and how I'd be filthy rich. I contemplated for a few months and in early January 2011 I decided that it was time. I loaded everything I had worth keeping into my 1997 no hub cap having, no radio, no windshield wiper motor, no trim, 8 mile per gallon Cadillac sedan hooptie and drove 11 hours to meet my friend with a self-tapper screw in my rear, driver side tire as a *plug*.

(This friend Nick Harvey, I am grateful for, if it weren't for him, this book wouldn't exist, nor would my life as I know it. My wife and children are in large part, because of his influence on me and my life. As I write this sentence it has been 2 months and 10 days since his death. The years that followed with him in this new working world I will never forget. Tales from our childhood through the end could fill the pages of another book. Good times and bad alike.)

The company housing where I would soon be resting my head turned out to be a 3-bedroom trailer with ten people living in it. My "room" was the kitchen floor. The work was incredibly arduous. We worked around the clock for what seemed like days on end. From one job straight to the next. I didn't mind much since I was there to make money after all. When we would finally get a few minutes off it was straight to the bar. We would drink anywhere that wouldn't card us because my friend and I were both still just 20. I hadn't outgrown the need for adrenaline, and I had taken about 2 weeks off from the lifestyle through Christmas and new year's before I left, so I was ready to go again. The living and working conditions led me and my adrenaline seeking habits down some twisted roads with some equally twisted people. Within 6 months of this new life, I had already put on about 60 pounds of undesirable weight, my inflammation was through the roof, and I felt like I couldn't do it anymore. I had been battling acne since my early teenage years and at this point it was damn near explosive.

The kitchen floor part was really wearing on me. I was wrestling the sand man for maybe four hours of sleep a night and getting woken up by other workers grabbing their lunch on the way out or grabbing food on the way in, it was relentless. Then there were the "visitors" to the house that had zero craps to give about me and my slumber stumbling around, sometimes literally stepping on me. I thought that the lack of solid sleep was the biggest issue making me so fatigued, so I mortgaged a home up the road. I was excited to sleep in a bedroom with a bed again. The partying and roughneck lifestyle didn't end there though so my exhaustion continued. Shortly after I turned 21, I hit rock bottom. I had been working over 100 hours a week for over a year straight, I was adrenally fatigued to the point that a six-pack of energy drinks a day, a bag of chew, a pack of smokes, and "other stimulants" were the only thing keeping me going. Oh, and all that money I was making, was wasted on keeping me wasted.

It was February in northern Pennsylvania, the coldest time of year. I had no money. I was working a long ways from the home I mortgaged and was working all these hours on what's known as a work over rig as a derrick hand, a fantastic position for the adrenaline seeking junkie I had become. The derrick hand works on the "monkey board" anywhere from 60' to 90' feet from the ground. I got to trip pipe, and swing around like a monkey rigging things up and hanging from great heights with nothing but a rope or wire holding me many hours a day.

The hourly pay was better (I think I was making 14 an hour), but I was still broke, and the calories from alcohol and energy drinks were no longer sustaining me. The illegal substances were barely even working anymore. This is when I really hit rock bottom. I was working about 3 hours away from the home I had mortgaged and couldn't afford a hotel room. I had recently earned myself a DUI, while I was sleeping in a borrowed car. I was tanked and in a "drivable" car, but I was sleeping in that car. The cops saw no difference and I believe they rather enjoyed detaining me. Despite my speed on foot and knowledge of the woods back home I had been in cop cars several times, but I would get dropped off somewhere with a good "talking' to" and "items" confiscated. It was a small town, I wasn't a bad kid, just did bad things and everyone knew it. I was one of the towns star athletes and my mom played a large helpful part in the community. She even made the cover of our local newspaper one time. It was an everyone knows everyone, and their out-of-state cousin's kind of town and the police never really wanted any trouble.

This was a new and different world though. I returned the borrowed car and got my truck to work. Started sleeping in it instead, only now I stopped getting tanked before falling asleep. I kept a pair of work bib overalls clean so that I could sleep in them and stay a bit warmer, kind of like a sleeping bag. I spent the rest of the winter going straight to a parking lot after work, avoiding my coworkers and wondering where I went wrong. How was I going to get out of this hole? How did I get into this hole? At this point in my life, there was no darker abyss, this was it. I was freezing my ass off every night trying to sleep in a cramped truck and working long hours in the freezing daylight. I was a day's drive from my family, a few hours from the shell of a home I had and those excess 60 pounds I mentioned I put on earlier were being broken down for energy. I went from a 170lb healthy(ish) minor league athlete to a 230lb drunk and then back down to somewhere around 160lbs. I quit drinking, smoking and the other illegal stimulants too. I couldn't afford them anymore, so quitting was easy. I was so fatigued mentally, physically, emotionally, and hormonally that I couldn't even think about chasing an adrenaline rush in any fashion beyond the rush associated with the nature of my job.

Winter ended, I finally had saved enough cash to stabilize myself, pay off my fines and quit the job. I found a more stable gig, less physical labor, and a slightly better schedule. As a plus I was getting a raise. The previous job was basically around the clock, I worked several hours before daylight until several hours after sun set 7 days a week. But this new job I only had to work 12 hour shifts 7 days a week. I was on the midnight to noon shift. An odd shift but I enjoyed it. I was able to sneak in close to 3 hours of sleep every night while on the clock, so I didn't need to sleep as much during my "off time".

I was still dealing with a lot of skin inflammation as this job started so I did a web search for natural ways to reduce or eliminate acne at a Wi-Fi hotspot-coffee-shop and it was recommended to eat avocados and expose my skin to as much sun light as I could without burning. My job required that I wear a hard hat, safety glasses, long sleeves, pants, boots, and gloves if I was working on anything. My face and hands were the only parts of me exposed to the sun. I would often hide out of plain sight and take off my hardhat and safety glasses and just stare at the sun through my eyelids. I bought a kayak and some running shoes to start really making changes on my off time. I was alone at this point, I worked as a one-man crew, had no roommates in the hotel, was far from home and the mortgaged home, at this point in my life, it was exactly what I needed. I didn't have a smart phone, computer, or any smart device. When I got out of work, I did one of four things. Went kayaking, swimming, hiking, or running. This routine lasted about 6 months. I didn't have any days off during this time, but it seemed like I never worked. My skin healed up quickly, I was able to maintain a decent four pack and I was figuring out day by day who I was deep down, and what I needed to do moving forward. When I was alone in nature, without any distractions, I would get into this flow state, like the "zone" that I had experienced in sports training and would just explore for hours. I thought I was exploring the wilderness but really, I was delving deep internally into my own soul. I was grounding while swimming and hiking (as I normally hiked barefoot), exposing my skin to the sun, exercising, and eating a little bit better without using stimulants I had regained about 10lbs and was back to a healthy 170lb. My life was turning around physically, mentally, and spiritually. I was seeing my self-worth again.

After working six solid months my supervisor asked me if I wanted to take a few weeks off. I had never been asked if I wanted time off before, so I said yes. I planned to spend a week in South Carolina where my parents and little brother had moved and then travel back home to Michigan for a week or so.

A year prior I had met this smoking' hot girl while out with a friend. We exchanged contacts but nothing happened beyond that. Never saw each other again, never even talked. Before the trip I went out and bought a small laptop and a camera. While setting up the computer I got distracted by social media (typical right?), I saw a post by that same hottie quoting John Lennon, trying to flirt through a screen, I commented. She messaged back, we exchanged numbers and that was pretty much the end of it. I hit the road running and set out to enjoy every second of my time off. I did, and somewhere in the mix I was wrestling with a friend of the family's kid, he snagged my phone and butt dialed . . . that hottie. I wasn't the nervous type. Not in high stake situations, not around women, not prior to a game, fight, interview, nothing, I just wasn't. But this girl, gave me the sweats. This impromptu butt dial sparked a fire that has burned hotter than a house fire in the Everglades mid-July ever since.

I returned to work with a re-found appreciation for life, I contemplated having someone to share it with. I started, as they say, "talk talking" to this perfect woman, and shortly after that I asked her to marry me. Today, we have three barefoot barbarians, a blue heeler, some ducks, a turtle, some frogs, and bunnies.

Once we got married, I got comfortable and started "fluffing" up again. The comfort led me back to chewing, drinking, and fighting. Just not as extreme. The job I had through most of this weight gain was an easy job, and the shifts were very inconsistent, sometimes I worked day shift, sometimes night shift, sometimes 24 hours. I spent a lot of time sitting and pressing buttons and this didn't help. The sleepless night shifts and 24-hour work shifts were stressing my body out once again, only this time I wasn't using stimulants outside of caffeine and nicotine. I was using a lot of energy drinks and sugary foods to keep me going and my waistline was the jiggly proof in the fatty pudding. We both had put on a few pounds, but mostly me. I was up around 300lbs. As a recap, I was a 170lb minor league athlete, turned 230lb chunky blue-collar worker, to a 160lb half homeless broken man, back to a healthier 170lb "found" naturalist, to a 300lb heavy weight all in a 5-year time span. This fluctuation was tearing my body apart at a cellular level and it wasn't getting better.

In the mix of this Kaitlyn and I knew that we wanted to start a family. We were both told at young ages for different reasons that our chances of conception were slim. We tried for a while and nothing happened, so we started to take our health a little more seriously. We didn't know where to start so we did the basics. More time outdoors, walking, and slightly cleaner eating habits. I started working out again, specifically running and we bought some home gym equipment. I didn't start losing any significant weight like that but I wasn't getting any fatter so it was a start.

In the spring of 2016, my wife and I found out that she was pregnant. The excitement couldn't contain itself, but something fired up inside of me that I had never felt before. I knew at that moment, as I looked down at my belly, that I couldn't raise a family in this state. I could barely bend down and tie my own work boots without coming up gasping for air. If I couldn't care for myself, how could I care for a baby? My wife knew the same, but we had no idea where to start. There is so much information about weight loss and fitness out there that it's a bit overwhelming. (As I add a book to that collection). During her pregnancy we began researching, while simultaneously cutting down on the appetizers, drinks, and desserts while continuing to spend more time outside and exercise a little. Kaitlyn put on some weight during her pregnancy but not nearly what she feared would happen (since every other mom out there was telling her to kiss her young body goodbye), and I had lost about 50lbs. The birth of my first-born daughter was perfect. She was as healthy and adorable as could be and we were so proud! At this point my wife and I had earned a few certificates. She had earned a holistic nutritionist and me a personal training certificate. Even in these courses, there was a lot of misinformation. But decoding this would take several more years of research and continues today.

The struggle was real. Like for real, real. For me, the reliance on substances earlier in my adulthood had taken a large toll. Defeating that demon was a serious battle and its outcome was a reliance on sugar, caffeine, and nicotine, in many different forms. Once I beat the nicotine and caffeine addiction it was just sugar. Which is arguably the most addictive "substance" on the planet. The opponent in this battle, although I often believe has been defeated, still has some rogue warriors lurking around that can come in strong with an ambush. Staying satiated has been the key. Adding to the struggle of change, working all hours of the day, sometimes working daylight hours, and sometimes working nighttime hours also created an alter ego I jokingly named "Midnight Trent" because of an insatiable Jekyll and Hyde like hunger craving that occurred in the middle of the night. It was relentless and always wanted something sugary, it took YEARS to resolve this and sometimes there is still a slight urge to wander into the kitchen around the time I take my midnight bathroom trip.

I dedicated myself to reading at least four books per month that pertained to health and wellness while continuing to better my body and regain my health. After about two months of this new dedication, we found out that we were expecting another blessing! Irish twins as they say since they were going to be under a year apart. My boy was on his way! My fire was stoked, as a father I needed to be able to play with them both, teach them, learn from them, protect them, support them, carry them, and most of all ENJOY them. I didn't want any activity to wear me out or make me say "no". "Daddy's tired" or "Daddy's sore" or "Daddy can't" even with my hectic work schedule I never wanted to be *too* anything to play with them. I wanted to be the father that could do it all. I wanted to be a good example of health to them. I had read a few books on epigenetics and although we had only changed our genes a little for our babies so far, we could help make sure that negative gene expressions wouldn't express themselves in them and then they could pass on better genetics to their babies and so on.

On top of that, I wanted to be the grandfather that could do it all. During this pregnancy Kaitlyn and I both focused much harder on our diets and continued reading and learning as much as possible. By the time my flawless son was born I had dropped another 30-40lbs. Still overweight but plenty happier and healthier than before. I was determined to take it to the next level. I am hanging around 180-195lbs of pretty-lean muscle. I'm happy, mobile, functional, active, inflammation is at an all-time low and I have never had this amount of control over my emotions and ego. I am more balanced and grounded than ever, and I am still progressing every day.

Throughout my journey I started helping men that worked the same way I did. Relentless hours, in hotels, all weather, all times of the day, lack of good food choices out of town, huge amounts of stress at work and from the house, and a surplus of other valid excuses to continue living unhealthy. I know the daily struggle of being a working parent, trying to supply an income, groceries, home, bills, love and affection for your spouse, children, family, home, and somehow yourself. It's a tough road, which means that you must WANT to traverse it. You will need to be extremely motivated to make the necessary changes. Find the fire that's in you, let that mother fucker burn hot as hell and don't let it cool down. What you do, what your genes express will become what your future children's genes express and their children. You are essentially raising your grandchildren. Don't mess them up. It starts with YOU, TODAY.

We pass on more to our children than we think. We pass on trauma, life experiences, fears, skills, passions, immunity, appearance, disease, or lack thereof, physical structure and more. What we pass on changes throughout our lives as our genes change. As we experience new things, in new ways, in good and bad ways we pass this on. That's the nature part of nature and nurture. This concept, once thought of as an either-or idea of determining behavior and traits. Genetics vs. the way someone is raised. Now is widely accepted that both nature and nurture contribute to one's behavior and traits. Our own attitude and behavior play a role in what genes will be utilized and expressed in our offspring as well. Our beliefs, our perceptions, and intentions shape our life all the way down to our molecular structure and function. Learning to control my "coping" mechanisms for those fears, angers, traumas, and life experiences, learning to beat that adrenaline seeking voice inside my own head, letting go of "triggers" and self-destruct protocols to manifest and create a better life was and is a long road to travel, but it is a glorious one.

For the average person there is a 66-day gestational period for creating new habits. Some people can develop new habits in just 18 days while others can take up to 200 days. This widely varying time frame is important to know as we look to create and maintain healthier habits, we must stay focused and see it through. Above all, we must WANT THE CHANGE. We need a valid reason to change, we need to recognize the cues, responses and rewards associated with the craving or habit so that we may make that change. Eliminating habits can be easier than creating new ones, done simultaneously though can be even easier. My inclination towards anger had become a part of me. I was addicted to the adrenaline rush I received for aggression, the situations in which anger is used and abused were adrenaline driven, and this led to addictions and other actions that further released these hormones, putting me in situations that were detrimental for my health and wellbeing. As a husband and father, I knew that this would affect my children long term if I didn't change it. I learned to redirect and harness these emotions in a way much more beneficial for me.

With my personal training clients we eliminate one destructive behavior or food ingredient per week and add one constructive behavior or ingredient. Taking small steps along the way choosing what habits we want to eliminate first and what new ones to incorporate. Slowly changing habits in a positive direction to ensure long term success is the key. "Inch by inch is a cinch. Yard by yard can be too hard." Jim Kwik, super genius, and author of "Limitless"

Consider the social acceptance and rejection associated with breaking and creating habits, consider if these social groups are good or bad for your change, consider whether they are supportive of your best interest and if they can remain a part of your life throughout your transformation. I lost many friends through mine. A bit through changing personalities and opinions, a bit through no longer having those same habits in common and a bit through spite. It will be bitter at the time, don't worry because it is worth letting them go. Unfortunately, you will likely experience this as you change as well. Don't let it get you down, jealousy and spite are self-inflicting weapons of hate, they will wish you ill so it's better to let those people go before they bring you back down. In the modern world there a multitude of things holding us from awakening the warrior the resides in each of us. You do deserve to be a warrior. Inside and out, you deserve to look like a warrior, defend, and protect like a warrior, pray, and meditate like a warrior, be as untethered, and free as a warrior, and to be as focused, and undismayed as a warrior, and above all FEEL like a warrior.

I have lived a unique life, as partly described above. As *un-holistic* and unhealthy a large portion of my young adult life was, I grew up in one of the most pure and natural environments in the United States. I have eaten many crayfish, freshwater clams, frogs, and a wide variety of freshwater fish over fires near the waters' edge where I harvested them, I have eaten venison backstrap, liver, and heart just hours after field dressing, I have eaten wild blackberries, mulberries, crab apples, paw paws, wild onions, morel and "white puff" mushrooms, mint from the waters' edge, and snacked on walnuts I cracked with stones in the woods. I worked several summers for a good friends' dad that owned a local greenhouse, I learned seed to harvest practices albeit on a small scale. I suppose that those humble beginnings called me back to re-evaluate my life after watching me stumble my way to rock bottom.

Today, my family and I grow an organic, compost fertilized, ladybug, and praying mantis protected garden that we eat fresh from and can from. We raise organic, free-range ducks for eggs. We sprout our beans, lentils, and chia seeds before we cook and consume them. Most of our food is prepared in our home on an iron skillet. I consume practically zero processed sugar. We pray as a family holding hands before we eat. We tell stories of our ancestors, souls, and magical creatures before bedtime. I push my body to its physical, mental, emotional, and spiritual limits as often as I can. We don't take any pharmaceuticals unless of course it's a life-or-death scenario. I do Wim Hoff breathwork prior to plunging into a trough full of icy cold water and meditate in a sauna several times a week. I do yoga both on my own and with my wife and family. I spend as much time barefoot as possible, and we sleep on a grounding matt next to a salt lamp and balancing chakra stone. We drink and bathe in filtered and mineralized water. I still read three to four books per month. I do Donna Eden's energy clearing practice daily. I developed a routine called the *Mindful Fitness routine* that uses my favorite energy stabilizing, strength building, balance, and functional movements without the use of equipment. A baseline energy warm-up from this routine is included at the end of the book. I love and live for my wife and children with more passion than anything in existence. We live the most holistic and sustainable way we know how, and all those epic failures led me here, to this new and improved life. I started as a warrior always looking for and creating a war. I have evolved into what I like to call a *Tranquil Warrior.* Knowing that I can enter any battle and succeed, but no longer searching for that battle in detrimental ways. The process is never fully complete because each achievement raises the bar another notch, I am thankful to be here for the journey.

Shall we get to it? Ah but first, a disclaimer, I am just a guy. I have no college degrees. Consult with your health practitioner before applying any of the methods in this book. The most relevant credentials I have are what you read in the introduction and that my wife and I are opening a soon-to-be successful fitness studio outside of Pittsburgh Pa. I am a personal and group fitness trainer. I played minor league football for two years out of high school. After that I entered real life, gained over 130lbs, fought with addictions, realized I was addicted to a lot more than I thought, fought with adult acne and constant inflammation. Lost the weight, added some muscle, managed the acne and inflammation. I worked my ass off for over ten years in the real world before finally deciding to follow my heart. I am a working father of three just like my wife who is my partner gym owner, boutique owner, a holistic nutritionist, yoga teacher, group fitness trainer, and reiki healer. I read and research a shit-ton. I exercise, I meditate, I use saunas and ice baths, I ground, I sunbathe, I laugh, and love. Over the years I have used myself as the experiment for all the practices in this book picking what works best for me, my wife, my children, and my clients. While minimizing time waste and frustration. It turns out that the most productive fixes in my experiences are paleo or ancestrally consistent which has led me to think mostly in this manner when it comes to human health. I am not a doctor; I am not selling you a special drug or treatment to magically fix your life. I'm just selling you this book. What you do with the information inside is up to you and only you. Please enjoy this book. And if you don't, feel free to put it down and give it to someone who will.

Blue-collar tips to fitness

I worked 100+ weeks for more than a decade, in all weather, surrounded by chemicals, high stress environment, out of town, artificial light through night shifts, all hours of the day, holidays, birthdays and more. The struggle is real as they say. As difficult as it may seem, fitness was still acquirable, and it is for you as well. I was notorious at the work site for having my cooler loaded down with "crazy foods", buying healthy lunches for the whole site, doing KB workouts at my tailgate, making bets on who could pick up heavy items on site, who could do more pushups or pullups and being spotted half naked, sunbathing behind my truck whenever I could sneak away.

There were times when I had been working for 30 or better straight days and no matter what I ate or drank, how hard I worked out or how much sun I got, I was still whooped, inflamed, and bloated. These are the times you need to prioritize sleep. I averaged 4 hours of in-bed time per day, maybe 3 ½ of that was spent sleeping. I started to really put sleeping in its rightful place and let myself take cat naps throughout the day, 5 minutes here or there when I could take breaks and ensuring I got to bed early enough. When I was still bright-eyed, and bushy tailed in the evening I would prepare everything I needed for the morning. Prepped lunches, coffee ground and ready to press a button to start the pot, to-go mug ready with some mushroom powder (typically lions' mane), to-go mineralized water, clothes on the counter, boots, keys, and hat by the door, truck fueled, and cooler loaded from the day prior. This way, I could wake up as late as possible before having to hit the road. Giving myself about 20 minutes to get ready at my own pace. After getting dressed I typically would do a set of pushups to failure and then twist and bend for a few minutes until my coffee was ready.

Key points to getting and staying healthier while working long hours in high stress environments. Prepare, set yourself up for success every single day. Sleep, quality over quantity but aim for at least 5 hours of solid sleep per night. Hydrate, with minerals and nutrients. Find somewhere to do pushups, pullups, air squats, lunges etc. while at the workplace and just rep out every few hours. Meditate whenever possible.

Awakening the Tranquil Warrior, All Rights Reserved. Trenton Sweet and Kaitlyn Sweet reserve the right to provide or deny use of any phrases or material in this book, written, recorded or otherwise. If you would like to use any of the work in this book or collaborate with the authors, please contact them directly through their Instagram social media platforms @The_Tranquil_Warrior (Trenton Sweet) and @Katies_Sweet (Kaitlyn Sweet).

CHAPTER ONE

DYING OLD AT A YOUNG AGE

"Many young men die at age 25 but are not buried until they're 75." Benjamin Franklin. What Franklin meant was that modern people let their joy, spontaneity, and love for life fade long before their physical body dies. This was not the case for our ancestors, nor does it have to be the case today.

We are often told that our early ancestors rarely lived beyond forty years. But that's not the whole story. This figure is thrown around like a solid piece of titanium but it's more like an egg. It is just an *average* life expectancy of a certain time period. Life span is how long a human can live; life expectancy is an average of a group of people. This average includes infant deaths, children, young men at war, slaves, young women during childbirth, people who were murdered or in accidents etc. Our early ancestors did not deal with the issue of war on the scale that we do today, nor the slavery, or murders. Unfortunately, pre agricultural humans dealt with a high rate of death from birth until teenage years, if a child could outlive these most fragile periods of their life, they could undoubtedly cruise into a ripe old age like one can today. Early agricultural civilizations were ridden with the same risks that hunter gatherers were but also dealt with the effects of war, famine, disease, murders etc. Rearing a child from infancy to adulthood was terribly difficult in the beginning of recorded history. As medicine improves so does the chance of survival during those fragile periods of infancy.

What about human *health span* and *health expectancy*? Health span is how long a human can remain healthy, as in free of disease, cognitive decline, tooth decay, disability etc. void of accidents and severe injuries. Health expectancy on the other hand is an average of how long the average human lives until their health begins to decline to the point of a disrupted life. It's no lie that "life expectancy" today is much greater (on average) than that of our recent agricultural ancestors. But what about our health expectancy and health spans? The CDC states that 26% of Americans have a disability (38.2% of which are obese as well), 51.8% of Americans had at least one chronic condition, and 27.2% had multiple chronic conditions (2018). The average age of Americans is about 38 years old. Over 41.9% of Americans are obese (CDC 2020), which is the leading cause of most of our country's ailments. But for some reason it is not considered a disease or disability. I wonder what the percentage of Americans living with some sort of disabling condition would be if you included obesity?

329.5 million people living in the United States in 2020, 85,670,000 have a disability, 170,681,000 have a chronic condition, and 138,060,500 are obese (going off of the percentages). That's a total of 394,411,500 people living with at least one health issue. Obviously, that can't be right since that's 70 million more unhealthy people than the number of people that live in the USA. What all that means is that most people with one diagnosed health issue, have more than just the one.

"Minor" as some of the chronic diseases may seem they are disabling and if they are not resolved and recovered from, they will undoubtedly lead to more diseases and discomfort. With an average age of under 40 years and the statistics listed above show that our health spans are declining as civilization "progresses". Our early ancestors experienced practically no disease or health decline. When a member of a hunting and gathering community would grow to an age where they began to slow, or weaken, the natural environment would eventually recycle them (as nature does). Compared to the way in which a modern human dies I would choose the quick and untimely predatorial attack over years and years of medicated decline. Modern humans suffer horribly the last few decades of their lives, kept alive, reliant on other people to clean them and move them around, barely managing their pain long enough to forget their own children's names. No thank you, that is no way to *live.*

Despite the facts, people today still believe that our quality of health is so much greater than our ancestors. I hear a lot of people argue against the paleo diet and lifestyle with the cliché "Yet, they died in their thirties." As we just discussed, this notion is based off average life expectancy and perpetuated by the medical establishment as stone-cold factual truth, they have twisted an average into a lie equivalent to a kid's story about how a ghost must've pooped in the bathtub, since they surely did not. When you know the truth, it's almost laughable.

Throughout history we have accounts of thousands of people both rich and poor living into their 100's. In Rome you couldn't even be a consul until the age of forty-three. People must have been living that long?! One consul M. Valerius Corvinos notably lived to 100 years. Augustus (Rome's first Emperor) lived to be 75 and his wife 86 or 87 years old. During certain eras it appears that the elites lived longer lives than did the poor but during others like the Victorian it is evident that the poor lived longer lives. The correlation between diet, time spent outdoors in clean environments, and manual activity are the difference.

Pre-agricultural revolution, archeological evidence shows extremely low amounts of disease and the degree of which is remarkably low compared to modern times. The carbon dating method is only good to about 50,000 years ago and hominin species have been around for more than two million years. Most evidence is anecdotal at best, no one had a birth certificate two million years ago, nor did they keep track of age in cave paintings. A look at modern day hunter and gatherer groups, a male once reaching the age of 15 can expect to live to 51-58 years but for a woman that reaches the age of 45 can expect to live from 65-67 years before their slight decline in speed, strength, vision etc. get them in a pickle. Noting health-span here, these hunter and gatherer elders are still as capable as many of their younger counterparts, performing daily tasks that far surpass what most seniors do daily in modern countries. In paleolithic times you must imagine humans being comparable to a wild animal. The young and old, slow and weak are always picked off first by predators, disease, famine, and incidents. Condensing the average age and limiting the length of life one could enjoy. But we can be sure that human lifespans are somewhere between 50 years and 75 years, and this figure doesn't seem to have changed much from ancient times through today even though our average life expectancy has. Many individuals today were brought into this world and kept alive with medical assistance and are lowered into the afterlife with additional support from medicine. Our lifespan has only artificially increased.

Our health span within the last three thousand years has declined, bone density has decreased, vision has deteriorated, tooth decay appeared, muscle strength declined, testosterone lowered immensely, estrogen increased, overall happiness has decreased, freedom has declined, labor has increased, and many diseases plague humanity that never existed before. But particularly over the past 100 years. The de-evolution that humanity was already facing, fast-forwarded with the advent of processed sugar, seed oils, EMFs, blue-lights, ungrounded and unnaturally padded shoes, clothing, intense all-day labor, harmful "cleaning" and "hygiene" practices, along with harmful chemicals and toxins in our food supply. Aren't we supposed to be evolving upwards? Sure, civilization has brought forth some pretty impressive inventions but what have we lost in the process?

We have lost our health, and our freedom, which are arguably the two most valuable things that a human has. Agriculture changed the way in which we lived communally. Hierarchies were formed in a way that limited freedom for anyone underneath the top of the totem pole. Today we are expected to choose a career while we are still young and then perform that career for our entire lives. This doesn't jive with the natural human spirit. Tribally, if you were an exceptional hunter, then you were probably expected to aid in hunts. If you were an incredible healer, you were probably expected to heal people. But you were not locked into this *job* for your entire life. People were truly free. Free from money, responsibilities, and materials.

Egalitarian bands of humans kept one another in check like a good crew of workers or family does. A hierarchy wasn't allowed to grow in a way where other members could be controlled by one or a small group of other members. When a member develops exceptional skills at something their head may begin to grow, if this happens, the rest of the crew/tribe knocks em' down a few pegs through hazing, joking, harassing and not giving them the credit that they feel that they deserve, this keeps any one member of the group from accumulating excess power over the rest, keeping the tribe more equal. While people with exceptional skills would've obtained great respect, they were expected to remain generous and compassionate, and not become a controlling entity. This is typical human nature, at the core of human psychology and sociology, we want absolutely no one to have control over of us in any way. This nature explains why people with healthier bodies, better hair, clothes, fame, fortune, power etc. in the modern world are roasted so blatantly on a regular basis. While today, this harassment doesn't necessarily keep them from having those things, it does rock their ego a bit and makes the rest of us feel better while taking away some of their power over us. Archeologists observing hunter-gatherer groups over the past few centuries illustrate in many writings this egalitarian approach to suppressing individual power while increasing group strength and cohesiveness well.

Hierarchies did exist but like in the animal kingdom they were fluid, meaning that no one individual could dictate what the entire tribe did for long periods of time. Any member would have been free to leave and join another group or go on their own whenever they pleased. Freedom contributes to health on a massive scale but there are more reasons why our early ancestors were far healthier.

When humans sowed their first seed our evolution shot quickly in a different direction and our health with it. We will discuss this more in a minute. What if a modern human with the help from medicine in times of trauma and emergency could implement the disease-free lifestyle of our early pre-agricultural ancestors? How long can humans we really live? People throughout history have pushed on into their 100s. A century is already possible, even before the advent of modern medicine and science. I believe combining ancestral diets, lifestyle, what we know now about quantum biology, and modern medicine that living beyond 100 is completely practical, 100 might even be a low bar. But we will have to tear down the system and the indoctrinated majority that is currently holding humanity back. How long do you think we could live healthily and happily without a debilitating medical intervention? I think a long time.

The Caveman's Quest For Satiety

Have you ever eaten an entire plate of nachos and were still hungry an hour later? Like you weren't satisfied? You should have been full right? I remember my days as a carboholic, I could literally eat 2 large pizzas, drink a six-pack of beer, and still feel like I could snack in a couple hours. Two large pizzas is somewhere between 4,000 and 5,000 calories, the six beers another 900 to 1,000 calories. In just one sitting I could consume about 6,000 calories and still be hungry in an hour! I don't know how this wasn't a *red flag* to me back then (the recommended daily amount of calories is 2,000 for the average adult). The reason why you still feel hungry after a subpar meal like that is because it provides minimal nutrients. Your body remains hungry because it still requires nutrients.

Satiety and being full are two different things. The idea of being *full* is ridiculous, we don't need to fill our stomachs to get adequate nutrition. Rather than filling your stomach you should aim for satiety. Which is the feeling of being full, like you have eaten plenty, even though you have not technically *filled* your stomach. Many people can sit and eat an entire bag of potato chips and still request a full-sized dinner but couldn't eat a 6oz ribeye, 4oz of bone marrow, 4oz of liver, and drink 2 cups of bone broth because adequate nutrition would have been achieved prior to eating that whole meal. Our ancestors knew the deal, fruit and mushrooms are a delicacy, meaning that they are enjoyable, but as far as nutrients go, they aren't optimal. They chose the most nutritious foods first and indulged in the other stuff when nutritional needs were met.

The human body requires 9 amino acids. Known as essential amino acids, or EAAs. These amino acids are easily acquired and digested through animal foods, although they can be found in plant foods it takes a much more deliberate diet with a wide variety of nuts, seeds, legumes etc. and will take much more eating. Avoiding anti-nutrients and plant toxins will require soaking, sprouting, fermenting, and/or cooking. Overconsuming many plants will result in gas and inflammation. When we don't obtain adequate amino acids and fats, we will remain hungry. The protein leverage theory states basically that until you've reached optimal protein (amino acid) levels you will still crave food. Meaning that whatever food is around, you will overeat until you've achieved the satiation of optimal protein, or you've literally filled your entire stomach and cannot fit any more food, in this case you will be hungry as soon as you have digested enough food to make room in your stomach for more.

In the world of nutrition there should be a substructure of micronutrients coming from each macronutrient so that people more fully understood where they should be getting their nutrients from. Micro-nutrients of protein would consist of your amino acids, fats would consist of the different chains of fats, and carbohydrates would consist of the different sugars and a sub-substructure for fibers. Not all proteins are created equal, not for humans anyways. We require the 9 essential amino acids in hefty amounts, we have huge brains, large bodies, large amounts of muscle, large capabilities, and large sexual organs compared to our closest relatives. We are an energy expensive creature. We live an extraordinary long time compared to our counterparts as well so let's take care of ourselves like nature intended and squeeze ourselves back into our place in the circle of life.

The human body turns macro nutrients like fat and protein into glycogen to be used in muscle action, but it cannot turn carbohydrates into protein or usable fat. Many people believe that you need carbohydrates to recover and perform well in competitive sports... I'm going to go out on a limb and say that our ancestral brethren that sprinted after a 3,000-pound horned beast with nothing but a sharp stick, launched it at them at full capacity, then ran it down until it was weak enough to attack again, then killed it, butchered it, and carried it back to their communal space a few times a week was 10x the *athlete* of any competitor today. They were likely at least 90% animal based and never thought to *carb load* before a hunt.

Amino acids are extremely important when it comes to cellular healing, growth, cognitive function, immune function, and muscular hypertrophy, something you want especially as you age, but there is one that stands out above the essential amino acids that is not considered essential. You cannot get this amino acid in plant foods; it simply isn't there. Known for its role in sports performance creatines muscular enhancement benefits have been recognized for decades. But it plays a huge role in cognitive function as well. If you choose to be a vegan, I highly recommend taking creatine and an essential amino acid supplement to ensure you are enjoying your most tranquil and warrior-like life possible. Also, these micro-nutrients of protein will make you feel full even after just handfuls of food. Eating less, fasting more is much easier when your body has what it needs to thrive.

From an evolutionary standpoint it's easy to understand why we become so ill after consuming copious amounts of *processed* sugar. The human gut evolved to digest a diet consisting primarily of meat, typically meat from ruminant herd species. Our stomachs are highly acidic for this reason. When consuming raw and potentially rotten or infected meat the gut must be adept in eliminating and neutralizing pathogens, viruses, parasites, etc. Our saliva serves as a "pre-digester", enzymes break down the food here first as we chew and swallow, once in the highly acidic stomach these potential threats are neutralized. This keeps those harmful bacteria invaders out of your intestines where they would have ample opportunity to reproduce and cause you discomfort and disease.

In a healthy human gut, you need not worry about this type of ailment, but when consuming a diet high in processed sugar, the proper acidity cannot be supported, opening the gates to harmful bacteria. Causing heart burn and acid reflux. As far as plant-foods are concerned humans in most regions had the choice of seasonal fruits, roots, nuts, seeds, herbs, and vegetables. Wild versions have shorter seasons, smaller yields, and lower sugar content whilst having a wider array of nutrients. Through much deliberation and communication from generation to generation the elders and experienced gatherers would teach others what plant foods were not deadly or harmful, and how to prepare them so they would be safer to ingest. They would teach which plants could be used medicinally or spiritually, which ones worked well together, which ones didn't, and which ones to avoid entirely.

Plants were on this planet roughly 100 million years before the first herbivores. Million, with an M, one hundred million years before herbivores. To put it plainly, plants are a step ahead of us. They developed a multitude of ways to defend themselves against would be predators and some plants found ways to use those "would be" predators to extend their own genes. I.E., bees, butterflies, moths, hummingbirds, and their relationship to the flowers. As well as every animal that consumes a fruit and then defecates its seeds in a pile of fertilizer away from the parent plant. And of course, squirrels and other animals that store nuts and seeds underground and then forget their location. Other plants, fungi etc. developed something even more special to the animal kingdom and humanity. By accident or purpose these substances have opened portals to spiritual realms otherwise difficult to find and traverse. Opioids, psychedelics, hallucinogens, and the like have attributed to the conscious evolution of mankind, without their use and implementation human consciousness would not be where it is today.

Co-evolution is the key here, when humans bastardized this element, our health immediately declined. There is ample evidence of this decline in archaeological data comparing hunter-gatherer communities vs. farming communities. When we began farming, we removed ourselves from nature, pitting us *against nature* instead of part of it.

Our first true ancestor moseyed their way out of the jungle about 2 million years ago. Evidence indicates that these early hominids lived primarily on small game, fruits, roots, nuts, seeds, and veggies prior to a climate change that decreased jungle space and increased grassland space forcing our ancestors out of the crowding jungles where our evolutionary path dramatically shifted. When they found themselves on the grasslands a few things must have become clear, small game was harder to catch, big game was harder to kill, predators were bigger and stronger, and we were the new species on the block, on top of those prolific odds the plant life consisted of mostly grasses. Adaption had to happen fast.

They stood upright to see out into the distance and over the tall grasses. Standing upright allowed them to use their hands more efficiently. They learned to move more swiftly on the ground, throw rocks and other "weapons" with accuracy, deal with hot direct sunlight by increasing melanin, reducing body hair to increase sweat glands, adapted to see movement more quickly, further away and peripherally, developed a keener sense of colored vision, and texture vision to differentiate edible plant foods and communicate through the whites of our eyes (a group hunting trait that allows fellow hunters to see precisely what the other is looking at without making a sound or movement).

Humans developed a smaller gut, a longer gate and increased mobility, our joints changed, and our brains and sexual organs grew vastly compared to our counterparts in the evolutionary tree. There isn't much debate over the mechanism that allowed for this quick and dramatic shift in evolution. Eating large fatty ruminant animals' nose to tail. Specifically eating organs such as brain, bone marrow, liver, heart, and kidney. All these organs are highly nutritious allowing our ancestors to spend nourishment on more "expensive" tissues and organs like our brains and sexual organs/attributes. Humans were scavengers in their new environment long before they were hunters. They likely watched the large predators go for the vital organs first (apex predators do this) and then eat the muscle meat last. Leaving the bones and skulls intact for our scavenger ancestors to crack open and enjoy. As evolution gifted them larger brains and increased hunting skills they learned and adopted the way of the apex predator, eating the most prized and nutritious organs first, continuing to consume the marrow and brains, working their way through the entire animal sharing their harvest with their entire tribe. Teamwork and survival became one in the same.

The level in which our ancestors were scavengers in the grasslands led to an even more acidic stomach than that of traditional carnivores because early hominins weren't just eating raw meat, they were eating raw meat that may have been sitting out in the elements for several days and picked at by multiple other scavengers and bugs. Evidence shows and modern humanity verifies that even after developing apex hunting skills, we still don't eat all the harvest fresh on the spot or even shortly after the kill as most carnivores do. We eat some now, some back with the tribe, some a few days later and some months later. Aged meat is a still a very popular food item today.

Early humans learned to harness fire at least 400,000 years ago (some estimates date past 1 million years ago) But to what extent these humans could build a fire and utilize it at-will is questionable. At whatever stage humans learned to harness fire successfully and repeatedly it was likely used for warmth, cooking, light, and defense. Cooking with fire opened the available food supply by a ton. The harnessing of fire undoubtedly led to the cooking of plant foods that had previously been difficult to digest, un-digestible or flat out deadly, cooking could break them down into a usable food. Cooking works as pre-digestion. Our prey, particularly the ones we evolved eating, have extra stomach chambers for breaking down plant food. We do not.

The amount of sugar consumed by early hominins is easily debatable, but the truth remains that it was far, far less than what the average American consumes today. www.dhhs.nh.gov states that Americans are consuming one hundred and fifty-two pounds of sugar yearly. That's roughly three *pounds* of sugar per *week*. In 1900, multiple articles claim different quantities, but they are mostly between one and six pounds per *year* of sugar. Yes, per year, the average American does that in a week. My great grandparents and grandparents despite living through famines and wars still managed to live healthily into their 80s and even 90s. Today, without medical assistance it's hard to say how many people can *healthily* live into their 60s. Diet, specifically massive amounts of processed sugar, play a massive role in this.

The Sweet Tooth Truth

Slavery and the acquisition of power make up most of the bitter history between our species and sugar, not so sweet huh? Processed sugar is now a multi-billion-dollar business making it one of the most powerful industries on our planet. Powerful enough to fund and manipulate colleges, politicians, scientists, media, and the like to maintain profits and acquit the industry from wrong doings. "Money equals power; power makes the law; and law makes government" Kim Stanley Robinson.

Sugar isn't just an American problem either; we may be number one when it comes to consumption, but we are not the only heavy hitters in this bout. Our neighbors Canada and Mexico are on the top ten consumers list too. Germany, Finland, and Australia are throwing haymakers as well. Humans crave and desire sugar more than any other substance. Our love of sugar has led to vile actions like exploitation, slavery, greed, genocide, and torture. But its havoc doesn't stop there, the biological damage its over consumption delivers also plagues us.

Sugar cane is a perennial grass. Humans are not equipped to digest grass!? It's true, grass eating animals have multiple stomach chambers to ferment, breakdown, and extract nutrients. They also have very resilient dental systems that help repair their teeth from the harsh minerals in grasses. Ruminants are mammals that chew cud regurgitated from its rumen. The rumen is the first compartment that receives food from the esophagus and begins to digest the food with help from bacteria, the ruminant regurgitates this cud, rechews it and sends it back to the rumen to be passed down the line for further digestion. Ruminants consist of cows, buffalo, sheep, goats, antelopes, elk, addax, deer, giraffes, yak, moose, and more, they have one stomach with four compartments: the rumen, reticulum, omasum, and abomasum. The ruminant stomach occupies almost three quarters of the abdominal space and is specifically equipped to turn grasses, leaves, flowers, seeds, and fruits/vegetables into nutrition. Human beings can eat grasses and not immediately die of course, but we are not equipped to extract nutrients from them, and the damages accrued in this attempt, make eating grasses a flat-out silly idea.

Do you know how many stomach chambers humans have? One. That's it, just one chamber that uses a churning action of the stomach muscles to physically break down food and releases acids and enzymes to chemically breakdown food. The stomach releases food into the small intestine in a controlled and regulated manner for digestion. Our colon serves as a fiber to nutrition converter, but archeology shows us that our colons have been shrinking ever since we left the jungles, further validating human transition from a plant-based omnivore to an animal-based omnivore. Most modern sugar as we know it today is a hybrid of several breeds of saccharum grasses or corn (which is a grass seed).

Processed sugar in general has no nutritional value. But particularly sugars coming from sugar cane and corn because they are both derived from grasses. Corn sugars I.E., high fructose *corn* syrup is potentially worse, just a theory of mine since corn is the seed of an annual grass, meaning that it is a highly protected part of the plant, plant-made toxins and chemicals (pesticides) are abundant in corn to insure its survival season after season. Annual plants are very protective over their seeds/babies, if they weren't, their species could die out rather quickly. Sugar cane is a perennial and is constantly bombarded by a legion of other addicted creatures, sugar cane is in defense mode all the time, meaning that it is always releasing defense chemicals.

Cane sugar was the first to be farmed somewhere between 8,000 and 9,000 B.C. the New Guineans were sucking the raw syrup from the cane and running small farming operations to harvest the sweet nectar. Similarly to how tribes farmed coca leaves for its neurological effects. These early farms weren't for a sustainable food source, they were for enjoyment. They ate the sugar cane raw, not processed. Just like tribal humans from all over the world (where honeybees exist) would eat raw honey from the hive, or maple syrup raw from the tree. As time went on these dense and natural sugars got processed until the side-effects far outweighed the "sugar-high". Do not confuse these processed sugars with sugars coming from fruits, honey, and maple syrup as there are digestible nutrients in them.

When consumed whole, fresh, and raw these sugars serve as adequate nutrition and energy.

Sugar cane was the bitter start of so much wickedness. It grows best in sub-tropical terrains because sugar cane needs a ton of sun and water. When the more *advanced*, modern civilizations caught wind of this liquid gold they opened sail to claim their fortunes. The Portuguese and Spanish started their exploitation on the tropical islands between Spain and the New world because of its perfect growing habitats. Sugar cane is the third most valuable crop worldwide. Projected to be a **90-BILLION**-dollar business by 2024. In 1492 Columbus sailed the ocean blue in search of spices. Sugar being among the most valuable and sought after, and that evidently holds true today.

Once civilizations got ahold of sugar there was no turning back. If they couldn't buy it, they would grow it themselves. Any plant that could be exploited and harvested for its sugar content was experimented with, each country in each climate eventually modified a plant to suffice their desire for sugar.

Processed sugar is hidden in almost everything today and has led humanity directly to several epidemics. The obesity epidemic, the heart disease epidemic, the diabetic epidemic, the mental health epidemic, the compromised immune system epidemic, etc. Sugar is one of the most destructive crops on earth. Whether it be sugar cane, corn (high fructose corn syrup), rice (rice syrup), sugar beets, or wheat.

Then why are we so addicted? Why do we CRAVE sugar so powerfully? If processed sugar is bad and natural sugars are good, then why don't humans just indulge themselves with some sweet fruit every day?

We evolved slowly on very little access to sugar. 15 million years ago primates experienced a mutation that allowed them to store sugar as fat more efficiently. This led to a craving for sugar in the form of sugary fruits, roots, and honey. No easy pickings' year-round though, this caused primates to seek out these foods whenever they were available. Remember though that these sugars our early ancestors craved were from whole foods, picked fresh, eaten fresh from where they had evolved to live, with the proper nourishment from the earth, climate, and sun. This craving never went away because primates that could more effectively store fat could inevitably survive for longer periods when other foods were scarce and developed a keener sense and deeper relationship with the available plant-food supply around them.

Although this evolution played a large role in our species survival, the sweet tooth adaptation sent humanity on a fast track to the agricultural revolution causing a huge problem for our future, and our planets future. Obesity is at an all-time high for adults, teens, and children. Now, this has become a problem that we pass on to our children and their children both through epigenetics and lifestyle. Increasing the intensity and severity of diseases each generation. Who knows how severe it can get if this continues? Obesity is both a precursor and an effect of the overconsumption of food, but most importantly an overconsumption of sugar. On top of that, our farmable topsoil has decreased from what used to be meters deep to just inches deep and requires supplemental assistance in most cases (unless farmed regeneratively). The biggest problem with processed sugar vs. natural sugar is that factory made sugars are much sweeter than their nature made counterparts making them more desirable to the human palate, whilst also being available year-round, inexpensive, and in an incredible abundance.

There is a direct correlation between processed sugar consumption and obesity. All-cause mortality is increased when an individual is obese. Cardiovascular disease is the leading cause of death worldwide, and you guessed it, being obese means you will most likely develop cardiovascular disorders leading to CVD. Worldwide obesity rates keep climbing and aren't showing any indication of slowing down as countries all around the world continue to load their plates and cups with processed sugar. Not only is processed sugar the most destructive substance to the human body when consumed in large amounts, but it has also had the most destructive effect on humanities interactions with one another and our planet.

I am not totally vilifying sugar, just the manufactured kind. Research indicates that humans do require a small amount of carbs for proper hormone balance and brain function. The brain DOES NOT require processed sugar. Eat your carbs in the evening and make sure they are coming from whole local foods void of processed sugars as often as possible. You don't need to hex the birthday cake at your kid's party, just use caution and ration. *Sugar hack,* in the case of a party or event, drink a tablespoon of apple cider vinegar (in a cup of water) before eating the cake. Many studies have shown that the apple cider vinegar lessens the blood-sugar spike and the impact from processed sugars.

Human Health vs. Processed Sugar

Consider the following statistics from the World Population Review 2021. 61% of adults in the country of Nauru are obese, 56% of the adults in the Cook Islands are obese, 55 ½% of adults in the country Palau are obese, 53% of adults in the Marshall Islands are obese, 51 ½% of adults in Tuvalu are obese, 48% of adults in Tonga, 48% in Samoa, 46% in Kiribati and Micronesia. We know that most people that suffer from obesity struggle with additional health issues, when looking at these statistics you should be shocked, and concerned. How did this happen to these people?

Nauru imports basically all its food. Which means that most of their food is processed and not fresh. NPR states that the main staples of the Nauruan diet are white rice, instant noodles, soda, and anything in a can. Anthropologist Amy McLennan told NPR that in the 11 months she lived there she was lucky to find one vegetable per week. Until the mid-third quarter of the 1900's Nauruan's still consumed an ancestrally consistent diet primarily marine life, fruits, roots, vegetables and coconuts (a fruit). But an increase in demand for the phosphate mined in Narau led to land destruction and economic advancement that made it increasingly difficult for locals to grow and sustain their own food supply and are now fed entirely by Australian imported goods. Nauru is the third smallest country in the world, yet it has the highest rate of obesity. The highest rate of type II diabetes, and unfortunately many people don't live past the age of 60. Genetically, until the mid-1900's the Nauruan's were healthy, active, and still practiced many of their ancestral traditions.

The story for most of the obesity stricken Pacific islands is the same, an exploitation of some sort of good that took up valuable food space on their islands taking away an ancestrally consistent way of living and eating. Leading to a reliance on imported food. Most of which being sugar laden processed foods like sodas, rice, and noodles. The dramatic and rapid shift in their economies decreased activity levels alongside the shift in nutrition but that is a lesser evil when referring to the obesity rate. Food is a primary cause. Lessened physical activity and the withdraw from tradition play a large secondary role. The food we eat connects us to our environment, and helps balance our energies, keeping us in the natural *loop* of our world, eating processed foods detaches us entirely from nature.

If we know how bad processed sugar is for the human body, and how rapidly it destroys human health in high amounts, then why don't governments and corporations put a stop or limit to its consumption? Why are countries that must rely on imported goods allowing their people to eat, suffer, and then die in this way? Why are countries that have an abundance of land and farming communities relying on processed food instead of real food? Why do governments allow heavy amounts of neurotoxic pesticides and earth destroying farming practices? Why do governments subsidize farmers to continue farming in such a way? Let's revisit the quote "Money equals power; power makes the law; and law makes government" from Kim Stanley Robinson.

The sugar industry is akin to the tobacco industry prior to regulations in this sense. The abundance of money made by the industry funds misleading studies and advertisements to keep the consumers believing that processed sugar consumption is safe and even beneficial. Next time you see a study about sugar having little to no negative side-effects take a deep look at who funded the study. You might rebuttal in Uncle Sam's defense saying that some government agencies have put out guidelines for individual sugar consumption, but we all know how far that goes. Especially when that same government putting a paragraph on a webpage or pamphlet to limit consumption simultaneously slams piles of sugary carbs and processed foods on our children's plates in our government funded public school system.

Who do you blame the dealer or user? In most cases we assume that the drug user "knows" the consequences of using the drug both on their body and legally. The dealer knows the consequences too, they share responsibility for the consequences as one cannot exist without the other. But what if the dealer knows all the risks and the user doesn't? What if there are no laws prohibiting its use and abuse? What if the dealer lies about the side effects? Or even convinces the user that using this substance is good for them? This is exactly what the processed sugar industry is doing. And what the tobacco, heroin, cocaine, and other substance industries/manufacturers did. Do a web search for old sugar adds and compare them to old tobacco ads, your mind might be blown. The street dealer is making thousands of dollars, but the sugar dealer is making billions. The street dealer will kill for their thousands, what will the dealer for *billions*? Which dealer is going to defend their business more diligently and to what extent will they defend their sweet devil?

The history of sugar is one of self-indulgence, gluttony, exploitation, and death. I won't sugar coat this, millions of people have been tortured, enslaved, kidnapped, extorted, exploited, and terrorized for its consumption by and for peoples ALL over our planet, no race, no religion, no region, no economic class is exempt from the corruption of sugar and the pain and suffering it has caused. Even the people that were being exploited would exploit other people, even their "own" people given the opportunity (Anthony Johnson 1620s, first recorded American black slave owner), this is how powerful sugar is. Sugar is highly addictive and if historical evidence of its destruction on our health and society doesn't convince you of this, I suggest reading all of Gary Taubes books, specifically "The Case Against Sugar", "Why We Get Fat", and "Good Calories, Bad Calories" and listen to the Great Courses lectures titled "The History of Sugar" by Kelley Fanto Deetz, you can also check out the work by TheSlaveRebellion.info website.

As stated earlier, sugar cane needs to grow somewhere sub-tropical, and takes a lot of labor to produce. Even today with all our modern machinery, boots in the dirt still toil and suffer to harvest this sharp leafed grass. The people that first exploited sugar cane for profit realized that they couldn't efficiently grow the crop in their native lands so they would need to exploit land in sub-tropical regions as well as people.

As the Spanish and Portuguese sailed the seas, they discovered inhabited and uninhabited islands perfect for sugar cane growth. This exploitation of land and people led directly to slavery on a scale much larger and different than previously known to humanity. Prior to this, slavery was primarily a punishment for the prisoners of war, thieves, and criminals. Captives would be sentenced to a term as a slave and would normally have a way to earn money and a way out *if* they survived their sentence whatever that entailed. Indentured was the term associated with this form of slavery. Often, they were permanently separated from loved ones and forced to assimilate into their new environment and punished severely for insubordination, but over all this slavery would have been an easier life than what this new crop would create.

Notoriously, slaves used by the sugar industry were treated extremely inhumane. As the kingdoms sailed around in search of spices, they found many nations at war in West Africa and islands with perfect opportunity to grow sugar. The nations that held prisoners of war were obliged to sell these prisoners for a profit. The sugar slave was a purchased slave. Not captured from an enemy. They were to be transported to remote islands or new lands that neither the owner nor the slave truly knew. This slowly abolished the *sentence* and chance to return home or earn freedom, the season after season work meant these sugar profiteers needed more and more consistent labor, plantation owners and government officials changed laws on slavery to facilitate the growth and riches the sugar industry was creating. These self-proclaimed *masters* needed non-stop slave labor, so much so that some plantation owners even tried to breed slaves for future use. But, since the living conditions were extremely difficult, the number of babies that made it through pregnancy to birth and then to adolescence was very low.

Today, those greedy people and corporations are still oppressing and torturing people. The torture now comes in the form of diseases, cancers, and a dismal destruction of genetic information to be passed on to the next generation. Escalating the extremity of these diseases and even new expressions of disease each generation. Have you ever seen a diabetic with missing legs? Amputation, is something that the masters used to do to their slaves... Harsh comparison? Maybe, but suffering is relative and all people on all levels of suffering deserve attention, disease and the internal suffering prior to appendage loss is indeed suffering.

An intense addiction to sugar

"Some studies have suggested sugar is as addictive as **cocaine.** People enjoy the dopamine release sugar brings daily. However, due to the addictive nature of sugar, long-term health effects like obesity and diabetes are a risk of its overindulgence. Like other compulsions or behavioral addictions, sugar addiction is a special risk for people with low moods, anxiety and stress." The previous quote comes directly from the Addiction Centers website. As always, downplaying the addictiveness of sugar. I have a few adjustments to make to the above statement. I would word it like this, "Many studies state that sugar is more addictive than cocaine and poses a larger-long-term health threat than do narcotics because of its social acceptance, celebration, and accessibility for peoples of all classes making it easy to overindulge in regularly. Unlike other addictions, sugar addiction is a special risk for every human due to our genetic compulsion to overeat and seek out foods that store easily as fat. Modern man is plagued with stress and anxiety, heightening that response to feast and store fat, making the abundance of sugar on our shelves a severe risk factor for billions of people." There, that's better. A true and non-biased statement.

"Sugar is noteworthy as a substance that releases opioids and dopamine and thus might be expected to have addictive potential." US National Library of Medicine National Institutes of Health. Again. I wouldn't sugar coat the findings here, if it releases opioids and dopamine then it has addictive potential.

I theorize that what makes plant-based drugs like tobacco so addictive might have a lot more to do with sugar than nicotine. At least the combination of nicotine with the sugar must cause it to be more addictive than nicotine alone, especially when you consider the way in which users of nicotine *administer* the nicotine, users smoke it in the form of cigarettes, let it soak through their gums (chewing tobacco), or snort it (snuff tobacco). These different administering techniques send the sugar and nicotine directly to the blood stream. The administration technique is a major factor when talking about a substance's addictive capacity. Sending it directly to your bloodstream is much more effective at getting those addictive chemical responses, because when you ingest something, your stomach does its best to break it down before sending them to your intestines where the substance is broken down more by bacteria and then gets into your blood stream. I believe that a direct shot to the blood stream of two dopamine releasing chemicals will surely lead to an addiction. Tobacco has a "nutrient" profile comprised of naturally occurring carbohydrates, or sugars that when used from the plant will induce a reaction like that of eating sugar. Adding to the addictive nature of sugar and nicotine, tobacco companies soak it in processed sugar before selling to the consumer. I was addicted to loose-leaf chewing tobacco from the age of 16 to about 26. I happened to run across a "sugar free" blend at a truck stop and thought "Hmm there's sugar in the other blends?" that answer is yes, a substantial amount when you break it down. Sugar works as a sweetener, a preservative and of course a way to keep consumers coming back.

A cigarette smoker consumes half a teaspoon of sugar per cigarette. Each pack has twenty cigarettes, that's ten teaspoons or almost one quarter cup of sugar per pack or about 42 grams. There is about the same in a pouch of chewing tobacco, each can of chew contains roughly eighteen pouches, the sugar content in each pouch is close to that of a cigarette and a can has about the same amount of sugar as a pack of cigarettes. Smoking just three cigarettes per day can increase your blood sugar levels by 29%. (HealthyDietforDiabetics.com).

Alcohols vary widely but some beers can have as much sugar as a can of Coca-Cola while most wines and hard liquors contain less. The average American adult according to USA Today consumes 26.2 gallons of beer per year (As of 2018). The average 12oz can of beer has about 11 carbs. The carbohydrates in beer are broken down into glucose so although the nutrition label says there is no sugar in your beer, those 11 or so carbs in your twelve-ounce brew are essentially glucose. Using the 26.2 gallon per year number, I broke that down to about two hundred and eighty 12oz cans of beer per year, per American. That's about 3,100 extra grams of hidden sugars per year. Or 12,400 calories. This number, due to a change in living conditions during the immune system crisis, has elevated to 28.2 gallons per year according to Beer Info and The Beer Institute.

Let's break down a bit of data. If you smoke a pack of cigarettes and drink three glasses of beer in one day you could be consuming roughly 75 grams of hidden sugar per day. That's 300 additional calories. Similar results if you chew a can of tobacco and drink a few beers daily. If you do this just five days a week you will have consumed an extra 1500 calories and 375 grams of sugar per week. If you do this 5 days a week throughout the entire year you will have consumed 19,500 grams of sugar and 78,000 hidden calories. And that's excluding 104 days from your year. Those 78,000 calories from sugar equal about 22 ½lbs of fat. When was the last time you heard of anyone adding a smoke or chew to their diet log?

The data in the last paragraph should make you wonder, with that high of a consistent sugar load, that when consumed releases opioids and dopamine, why is nicotine the substance vilified? 40 million Americans use a tobacco product daily. Alcohol has no nicotine, or any other addictive agent besides that contributed by sugars. Yet alcohol is listed as the second most addictive substance. Nicotine is listed as the fourth, but sugar somehow misses the addiction centers list all together.

According to WebMD, scientists have done numerous studies to determine why alcohol is addictive. The studies proved that **alcohol primarily affects the reward center of the brain.** When a person drinks, endorphins are released. The more a person drinks, the more endorphins are released, according to the study. But what causes the endorphins to be released? Doesn't there have to be something in the alcohol, some trait associated with the alcohol that reacts with your brain and hormones? Is it one of these sugars like erythritol, glycerol, lactitol, maltitol or ethanol? Ethanol appears to be the sugar that makes you feel drunk, which can be an amusing component contributing to its addiction. But each sugar helps to play a role in releasing those addictive endorphins.

Sugar, particularly those naturally occurring in fruits play a role in proper brain function. Compared to what most Americans would consider a normal sugar intake the amount necessary is very low. There is a large difference in the way in which your body uses the sugars in an apple compared to the way it uses the same amount of sugar from a soft drink. Isolating sugars and manipulating them to add to foods in un-balanced and unrecognizable portions complicate the way it effects the body. An in season, naturally ripened apple for example contains about 60% fructose, 20% glucose and 20% sucrose. High fructose corn syrup on the other hand is 55% fructose and 45% glucose. Naturally occurring ratios make whole foods delicious and nutritious. But secluded, manipulated, manufactured, processed, and mixed in unnatural ratios turn a once nutritious source of energy into a harmful substance.

Gamma-aminobutyric acid (GABA) is a natural chemical produced by the brain. It is a valuable anti-anxiety neurotransmitter. When we experience stress, the adrenal glands are prompted to produce hormones that trigger what are commonly known as fight-or-flight responses, like speeding up your heart rate or giving you an adrenaline rush (WebMD's definition). When an individual has low GABA production they regularly suffer from anxiety and depression. When consuming low amounts of sugar, GABA is released to reduce excitability from the sugar rush. This is normal. When consuming excess sugar (especially processed sugar), GABA production is decreased, causing an elevation in excitability leading to anxiety and depression. If left unchecked, this underproduction of GABA can interfere in one's social life, serious side-effects like suicide are commonly reported when a person becomes chemically imbalanced. A direct relationship between insulin resistance and decreased GABA production exists, although the precise mechanism is currently unknown.

CHAPTER TWO

USING ANCESTRAL WISDOM IN THE MODERN WORLD

I believe in eating a diet as close to our ancestors as possible and yes this does imply that some of our ancestors ate differently. Evidence suggests that all human beings originated from Africa around 2 million years ago. Evidence also suggests that early humans began adventuring the world shortly thereafter. Fun fact, the oldest pyramids in the world are found in the Americas. Yup, that continent that was coined "The New World" was truly the old world. Humans that travelled the world evolved and adapted separately to different environments as they explored. These environments, despite the obvious differences of climate and terrain also contained different food sources. If you know your family origins, then you have half the data needed to understand what diet will be the most consistent to your genetic makeup. I say half because when you take most ancestry tests you are shown a country or region of origin that only dates back a few thousand years. You will need to dive a bit deeper and uncover where your family may have traveled from, before settling in the presented origin. My ancestry shows strong Scottish, Irish, and Northern European roots from both my mother and fathers' sides. I know that Northern European settlers from the times before agriculture were nomadic and had most likely spent a lot of their evolution in the space between Northern Asia and Europe. These people were known is early

Eurasian hunter gatherers. For me, researching this region and the food sources available between 20,000 and 100,000 years ago gives me the most ancestrally consistent diet for me personally. You are different, as all of us are so do some digging and find out what works best for you. You might uncover that your ancestors indulged in plenty of raw dairy but when you try to incorporate it, the reactions are less than satisfactory. Humans exhibit a wide variety of biodiversity, to square it up perfect for you, you'll have to experiment.

Implementing light fasting and eliminating sugar can be difficult when raising a family. Trust me, I know. Especially when your mother in-law owns and operates a superb bakery. Our children still get Grandmas treats from time to time but at the house the only options are healthy options.

The kiddos request pancakes and waffles for breakfast a few times a week, under normal conditions we would say "No" but since we home-make them it's a fun way to sneak in minerals and nutrients. We use a paleo mix, that seems to make the best tasting waffles and pancakes with the least garbage, we add things like fresh and fertilized duck eggs (from our own free-range ducks), grass-fed and finished bone marrow, and organic bananas or pumpkin to the mix. They get their "treat", we get the satisfaction of knowing its healthier than the average pancake. If they request "syrup" they normally get raw, local, organic honey. If we are feeling wild, they will get some local, organic maple syrup. They drink water with a few drops of trace minerals. NO JUICE unless it is a very special occasion. The older they get, the more solidified their eating habits will be, so start making the adjustments necessary now. Think about how hard it is for you as an adult to make consistently healthy choices, don't let your children fight the same fight. Our trick with the kids is to let them snack on whatever they want and help decide what to make for meals. We do our best to only keep items in the house that we are okay with them eating regularly.

Let your children grocery shop with you, let them pick out what they want if it fits your objectives of course. If they insist on a certain snack that doesn't fit the guidelines, then find something similar that does or make it yourself. Raising kids in today's world boils down to making the best choice you can at the time. My wife makes marshmallows, brownies, cookies, hot chocolate, and a plethora of other sweet treats at the house. She uses better paleo ingredients to stay true to our goals, this lets them enjoy treats of the modern world while staying healthy. Your kiddos taste buds will adapt. I promise. Their health and attitude will improve. The secret is, they *must* see you eating the same foods. It cannot be a "diet" for you and especially not for them. This is psychologically backwards and will not permanently change anything for the better. Don't create a bad relationship with food just create a NEW relationship. One that reconnects you and your family to ancestral traditions and nature.

Our children snack on jerky, cheese, yogurt, carrots, and fruit from dusk 'til dawn I swear but they also eat a decent portion for breakfast, lunch and dinner. Again, letting them choose. Another sidenote here as far as raising tranquil warriors, don't *make* them finish their plates. This was hard for me. I was raised to finish my food before I could leave the table. I used to get so frustrated with the kids for not finishing their food. It isn't worth it. If it's a meal that they chose, both out of the fridge and from the grocery store they are more likely to finish it at mealtime and if they don't, it's okay. Children won't overeat nutritious food. Just like an adult, once your body has what it needs you will feel full. Try overeating something like liver or bone marrow, I bet you throw in the towel long before you have consumed as much is necessary to "fill" you up if it were pizza instead. If your kids aren't finishing their plates, there is probably a reason. I will say though, saving that plate for later may not be a bad decision if their plates remain full after mealtime. No one wants to see good nutritious food go to waste. Leftovers will mold, even after a day or so, try not to eat leftovers that have been stored for longer than two days.

Dinner is the feast in our house. We strive for an earlier dinner like 5pm in the winter months and 6-7pm in the summer. This isn't always possible, but it is the goal. The earlier the better, preferring 4-6 hours before bed. Everyone eats as much as they desire, once everybody's food has settled and the kitchen/dining room is all cleaned up we normally play as a family until bedtime. Then we read a few small books, tell some stories, say our "I love you and Good nights" and then its sleepy time.

Karma and the Carnivore

Humans evolved to consume animals from nose to tail as a primary fuel source, enjoying fruits, fungi, and other plant foods as "side dishes" and survival foods. This animal-based ancestral concept goes against a large portion of today's *health enthusiasts.* As a vegan or vegetarian, you need to ensure you are getting adequate minerals, vitamins, and nutrients or else your health can decline in the long term and your children, and their children will undoubtably see the effects of this malnutrition if you serve them the same diet as yourself no matter your love and compassion towards nature. For anything to live, something must die. Whether what dies is a beet or a bison. In terms of the actual animal death toll when looking at animal based vs. plant based believe it or not, farmed plant foods pile them higher. Modern farming practices kill millions of creatures like worms, weasels, moles, mice, rabbits, toads, turtles, squirrels, snakes, and many more are tilled to death. And that doesn't include the native funguses and plants. Their habitats are ripped away and whatever animals manage to survive the till and clearing are killed by the farmers or pesticides. Home grown gardens and/or regeneratively farmed is the best way to choose any food item, because this practice allows for more of what nature intended.

Through my wife and I's spiritual journey we have come across and become good friends with dozens of vegans and vegetarians that have chosen this path for many different reasons. Some have chosen it because the government says it will fix climate change, some because the government says that meat is bad for you, some to signal their virtuous ego, some of them that avoid politics have removed animal foods because they believe it gives them more spiritual abilities, makes them more open etc. It is believed that meat takes a lot of energy to digest and therefore wastes energy that could be spent elsewhere. As we discussed earlier the human gut and digestive system is designed to digest meat, less designed to digest meat covered in spices and cooked to a crisp. Difficulty in digesting spicy, over-cooked meat is likely associated with this connection between digestion and energy consumption. Others do it strictly for the sake of karma. This comes from the idea that not eating animals means that you are not contributing to the death of anything. That isn't just wrong, its dead wrong. The soil has been so depleted and removed from its natural cycle that it needs *fertilized*, which is done using bone meal (the bones of thousands of animals for minerals), blood meal (the blood mixed with other compost for minerals and nutrients), and fecal matter from conventionally farmed animals. Sounds like a death toll to me. I understand the concept out of sight out of mind, it's kind of like watching it rain cats and dogs outside while looking out your kitchen window, but then you turn your back away from the window and say, "It isn't raining." Even though it is raining, you aren't seeing the rain, so you aren't wrong in changing your perception, but the truth is, it's raining. Turning a blind eye doesn't make you a saint.

Shame and guilt have no place on the road to awakening your tranquil warrior. I don't make you aware of these misconceptions to make you feel ashamed or guilty, I used to believe the propaganda too. I hope that you may see the truth and move forward in a more productive way. Something living must die for something to live. That is the cycle of life, everything is born again. Pretending that you are better than somebody else because of a preconceived lie does not make you a better person. It makes you an egotistical fool and separates you further from nature.

Does the wolf suffer from the effects of karma because of its carnivorous ways? A lion or lioness? Does a pod of dolphins accrue bad karma when they murder a great white shark? Does an eagle or hawk collect negative karma when it brutally snatches up a cute little bunny and serves it live to its hatchlings in the nest? What about an ant eater when it sucks half a colony of unsuspecting ants from their homes? Or how about a group of panda bears when they devour a forest of bamboo? Or what about a Venus fly trap when it consumes a fly? One more, what about when a mushroom infects an insect and turns its living body into its new home, killing the bug in the process? I had this conversation with a 5-year vegan on a worksite recently and he informed me that those were irrelevant questions because only humans make conscious decisions. I said "What? Wait, so humans are the only conscious animals on the planet? And that consciousness brings with it both good and bad energies that can influence our existence for infinity?" He assured me that yes, only humans have this trait. Now, I am no saint, nor would I even consider myself a good example of having great morals, but this has never jived with my understanding of life. We may be the only animals that feel guilt and shame on the massive and long-term scales that we do, but we are definitely not the only species with a conscience. Two sayings come to mind when I hear arguments like this, *ignorance is bliss* and *out of sight, out of mind.* Plants communicate and cooperate much more efficiently than humans do, they can care for, share with, and communicate threats to a plant of another species many miles away from them through the fungal networks in the soil and chemicals *scents* in the air. Just because our sense of perception is different doesn't mean that these living things are not making conscience decisions.

Civilization led us to create polarity everywhere we go, us vs. nature, positive and negative, right and wrong, we love to divide things, like "animals have souls but nothing else that is living." A common belief is that animals have souls, but maybe not birds or fish, or even reptiles. So, what, just mammals have souls? What a preposterously egotistical idea! I used fancy words there to emphasize the ridiculousness of the idea.

Our ancestors knew that we weren't so special or separate from everything else, even elements and minerals that modern science declares lifeless were given spirit and energetic forces. Plants, mushrooms, and algae have energy, spirit, and/or soul as well. They are living. Mushrooms were here before plants; plants were here before insects, and the rest of the creature kingdom so what makes the life of a buffalo more significant than the life of a shiitake or a carrot? I believe that ego is what makes some lives more significant than others. As hard as it might be to grasp, humans are a part of the circle of life. For us to live, living things must die. When we die and if we choose to be buried, we will be consumed by insects, fungus, plants and maybe animals as well. Those living entities will all die one day, and the outcome will be the same for their remains. This is the circle of life. The further that we separate ourselves from it, the further the circle of life separates itself from us. And *that* I believe is where dis-ease truly begins. We are the only species on the planet that doesn't *know* what it is supposed to eat. We separated ourselves from nature. I have always seen God (by whatever name you prefer) as nature. And nature can be seen as... everything in the infinite universe. If you are separate from nature, you are separate from God.

Hominins lived off consuming mainly ruminant species, other animals, some mushrooms, and fruits for more than a million years and our health was undeniably fantastic. After the agricultural revolution when humans began eating plant foods in abundance our health began to decline and has been slowly declining since. With the obvious introduction to processed sugar being one of the most detrimental additives. There are a multitude of nutrients that only come from animals, and/or come in much more bio-available forms and in larger amounts in animal foods. Meaning you can eat much less on an animal-based diet and get more nutrients than when eating a plant-based diet. People still claim though in the face of mounting evidence that they prefer to be plant-based. If you are one of those people and prefer a plant-based diet I recommend reading Darin Olein's book "Super Life" and take his advice on eating a very wide variety of plant foods, fresh, local, organic, and in-season. Sticking to your guns is great, just don't hang on to that trigger so long that you miss-fire and shoot your own foot. The ancient cultures of enlightened people that didn't eat *meat,* got the powerful animal-based nutrients from foods like ghee, butter, tallow/lard, raw milk, cheeses, and eggs. Track your intake to ensure you aren't missing the mark on nutrients if you choose to avoid nose-to-tail nutrition.

Americans have been "plant-based" for a few generations now as the government has recommended that we consume massive amounts of carbohydrates primarily from processed grains and cereals, including the plant-based motor oils they claim are *heart healthy*, and minimal amounts of animal-based products. Many of these ideas were first initiated by John Harvey Kellogg, yes, that Kellogg. The same one that created the still powerful propaganda that breakfast is the most important meal of the day, which was created as a slogan to sell his products. John and his brother Will Kellogg created cornflakes with the intention to stifle sexual drive. Kellogg's propaganda is still believed and taught today, for example self-pleasure or masturbation (which is plenty more natural than many believe) was an awful sin, one that led to many ailments and potentially hell, he wrote of many ways to ruin sexual pleasure for both men and women alike. The whole *coffee will stunt your growth* thing, also John Kellogg, because coffee offers a stimulation that provides pleasure, and pleasure, was bad according to the Kellogg idealism. Kellogg believed that REM sleep was something to be aware of as well, calling it a curse of a disorganized and polluted mind. He claimed that natural sleep should be dreamless, and consciousness entirely suspended. He is also to blame for many disturbing ideas to deter a young child from touching their private area, which he had created a large list of behaviors in a child that proved without a doubt that they were sinning in such a way, including bashfulness, boldness, bedwetting, lying, and trouble in school. Behaviors that most children exhibit at one time or another. He developed and instructed ways in which a parent could *justifiably* keep their child from sinning. Bandaging of the parts, tying the hands, or covering the area with a cage. Sometimes that wasn't enough so of course the next option is to cut off a large portion of the male's sexual organ, a practice that you are frowned upon for pondering the efficacy and morality of today even though it is still practiced, circumcision. Done without anesthesia because the pain would work as an additional deterrent. For the girls, an even more vile approach of cutting off the clitoris and labia minora was the final attempt to *save* them from *self-abuse* as he called it. The worst part about this cynical man's ideas was that he truly believed he was doing right in the name of God, he was a glorified doctor and people trusted him deeply. Yeah, disgusting I know. This is the guy whose ideas and propaganda supplied governments with the *facts* that later created the food pyramid. That is reason enough for me to ignore all those recommendations.

Society pushes each year for additional plant-based products and each year human health declines with it. Lowered libido means that there is a damaged endocrine system. Consider this, cheesy puffs, popcorn, captain crunch cereal, and little Debbie's' are plant-based.

As our soil disappears and our planet grows increasingly sick, it is more important than ever to seek the truth and eat regeneratively. For the planet's health and yours, organic, pasture raised, regenerative, 100% grass-fed and finished, and non-GMO are utterly important, those labels ensure the best for our internal and external environment. As well as for the lives being consumed, animals and plants. Modern day, conventional farming is highly destructive to our planet, the lives being consumed, and our health. Choose no-till if you can and always local. When hunting and fishing, eat what you hunt or catch from nose to tail, honor the animal for its life and thank nature for her bounty. The spirituality and connection to nature through hunting and harvesting your own food is unbeatable. Not to mention the nutrition. Don't believe the stereotypes, most hunters that I know (even some heinous ones) pray in some way over their kill, thanking it for its death. As I like to say, pray for your prey, it is nature's way. Hunting, fishing, and harvesting are similar in this way. Any life taken purposefully to sustain another life should be thanked and gratitude given. With respect we eat and use as much of its physical body as possible.

Today, giant corporations that essentially run our government and media are pushing that Americans eat less of the healthiest foods on the planet and more of the factory-made and least healthiest foods. Producing foods that are good for humans' cost more and have a lower profit margin compared to factory-made "foods". A few things come into play here. One, factory made "foods" have a longer shelf life, meaning that there is less waste and more profit. Two, they are extremely cheap to manufacture. Three, factories can produce massive amounts of these "foods" in a short amount of time. Four, because of the extended shelf life these products can be made in countries with little to no labor laws and then shipped to the U.S., bringing overhead costs way down. Five, all the reasons above increase profit. If they can convince the whole world to eat in this manner, they can increase profits even more.

The capitalist billionaires that so many people claim to despise are the ones pushing the plant based, (I mean *plant* as in factory) factory-based diet because it will make them significantly richer. The push is hidden behind a shield of "we care about the planet" and "eating animals is mean". But it's just advertising. Good advertising, as it touches people right in the feels. Climate change is real, but humans have contributed to it, not caused it. We cannot just stop doing what we are doing and stop climate change. It will happen, nonetheless, even if the entire planet switches to electric everything (most of our electricity is generated by natural gas, coal, or nuclear power plants anyways). And as it gets hotter the earth will not die. Our destructive farming and manufacturing practices will destroy her but not climate change. We are coming out of an ice-age and the periods before the ice age were much warmer than it currently is. During the Cretaceous period where a plethora of life from all kingdoms roamed the earth there was no ice at the poles. Life was abundant. Stop freaking out, stop letting these rich giant corporations bully you.

Some sub-groups or religions over the last few thousand years have been able to thrive on mostly vegetarian diets with minimal meat consumption. I argue that dairy and eggs helped them maintain their vitality, but the point is that they did thrive. And that's a valid argument for today's vegetarian. But these people were not vegan, or *plant*/factory based. It's important to know that being a vegan or vegetarian in the modern world is massively different that it was a few thousand years ago. Our soil is all but depleted of nutrients and minerals due to harsh farming practices. Meaning that the plants we eat today, organic, or non-organic have *far* less nutrients and minerals than the plants our ancestors consumed. Human biology has been losing a bit of resilience every generation since the agricultural revolution and as this decrease in vitality progresses it also multiplies in intensity. Today, more nutritious foods are essential, unless of course you wish to become the humans in the Disney Film WALL-E. Growing your own organic garden with a large variety of plants, using organic compost and minerals is a great start to reclaiming your life force if you choose to avoid animal products.

What "tag" is the best bang for its buck? Is there a "Catch all" label you can see and just know that it's the best of the best? What all labels are out there? These are popular questions I get from clients, and for good reason. No one has the time to decipher every ingredient and label when they are shopping. Here's some common ones, organic, non-GMO, fair trade, sugar-free, zero calories, local, 100% grass-fed, grass-fed and finished, pasture raised, cage free, regenerative, vegetarian fed, etc. There are so many labels to look for. As far as looking at meat labels goes, understand that cage free does not mean free to roam or even that they are raised outdoors. It simply means that they don't live in a cage. They could live in a barn, on cement, surrounded by a million other animals, they just aren't in a cage. Organic means that they were fed organic food, it says very little about the living conditions. Grass-fed could mean that they live their whole lives in a stall and are fed grass, but it doesn't mean they ate grass their whole lives, they could have had just a few meals of grass. Grass-fed and finished means that they ate grass their entire lives, which is more ancestrally consistent than typical cattle feed, but they may still have lived in a stall. Vegetarian fed is a tricky one, if you are buying rabbit meat then sure vegetarian fed makes sense but not if you are buying chicken or chicken eggs. They aren't vegetarians, so that means they aren't eating a diet that is consistent with their biology, meaning they are sick and inflamed. What you really want to see are labels like, organic, pasture raised, grass-fed *and* finished, non-GMO, local, and regenerative all in one if possible.

When looking at plants and funguses you'll see a lot of the same labels listed previously but the best bang for your buck is going to be organic. This label guarantees a minimal use of pesticides and chemical fertilizers while also being non-GMO. Plants die after they have been removed from their life force, so it makes sense that some of that life force that we call nutrients would start to slowly decrease as it was trucked to your store. Choose locally grown when possible. Choose organic and scour the racks for regenerative.

When looking at packaged goods (which I hope you don't buy bulk in after reading this book) avoid products with long lists of ingredients, period. I could list all the deadly chemicals that are in our foods today, but it would fill several pages. Fewer ingredients are always better. If you see hydrogenated oils, any seed oils, artificial flavors, artificial dyes, processed sugar, or carrageenan put it back on the shelf. "Zero sugar" or "zero calories" and "low carb" don't mean that your body won't respond to those ingredients the same way that it does to "real" processed sugar, carbs, and calories. Because it does. To boot, the sugar that's in those sugar free and zero calorie foods and drinks activates hunger hormones making you hungrier later, especially for sweets, and promotes fat storage and gain. Sucralose is the culprit you will be looking for on those labels.

Back to that "catch all" label we were looking for to make your shopping experience easier. The label is increasing in popularity but is still pricier than average products because of its rarity. The more that the whole world understands this method and invests in it the cheaper it will become. Regenerative. This label guarantees that animals live outdoors, free to roam in adequate space, eat an ancestrally consistent diet, and the practices used to farm both animals and plants are benefiting our planet. A truly regenerative farm doesn't till the land because this kills millions of microbes, small animals and bugs and depletes the soil of carbon, a regenerative farm allows their livestock of all kinds to range free upon plentiful open space similar to their natural habitats with their ancestrally consistent diet available for grazing, they utilize their ability to turn food into fertilizer and once they have eaten down a good bit of the pasture they move them to another range, moving in another livestock behind them or planting a crop in the freshly manured and cleaned up field. Soil never gets depleted (in fact, more is created), the animals are happy, raised to a peak age, mothers allowed to raise their young, males and females alike are allowed to breed and play as they would in the wild before being humanely harvested or hunted on some of these farms, plants grown in naturally fertilized soil devoid of pesticides contain more nutrients, since the soil is healthier it retains water much better, meaning the crops need much less outsourced water to produce, and this style of farming sequesters more carbon into the soil (where it belongs) than is used during the operation. Meaning that regenerative farming is carbon negative, reducing its footprint into the negatives, where conventional farming methods release massive amounts of carbon into the atmosphere where it contributes to global warming. Eating in this way will reconnect you to nature, and assist in the awakening of your tranquil warrior as it realigns your energy in a natural way. Read the book "Dirt to Soil" by Gabe Brown for more information on regenerative farming.

Hunting and gathering with a shopping cart

While navigating our strange new world where most of our foods are made by giant corporations with zero interest in health and 100% interest in profits it's hard to decipher what foods are nutritious and what foods are poisonous. In nature, there are signals to which foods are edible and which are not. In nature something poisonous might have a burning, itchy, or poky feel, maybe it tastes awful, sour, bitter, spicy, or numbing on your tongue. It might have an irritating smell or make your eyes water just being near it. If it's a fruit that isn't ripe it blends in with its environment, it turns a more vibrant color when its ready. In the grocery store, where modern humans "hunt and gather" everything is made to look, feel, and smell edible and extremely palatable. Foods are presented in packaging that makes us hungry and has blatant lies all over the product. When you look around the store your hunger creeps in and next thing you know you've put 30,000 calories worth of processed sugar and poisonous chemicals in your cart! They design modern foods with this intention, profit over health. Some people think "Hey, we have the FDA that protects us from harmful ingredients in our food.". Read Vani Hari's book "Feeding You Lies" and you will become aware of how heavily this administration is funded and influenced by the same companies manufacturing the poisons that they are supposed to be protecting us from. Part of the awakening is understanding your role and responsibility.

Knowing the truth will awaken your ability to be a tranquil warrior.

Other countries around the world, even "third world" countries have banned thousands more ingredients than the FDA has. The FDA is aware of thousands of ingredients that have mild to severe side effects but do nothing about it. The proof is in the pudding, and the jello, and in pretty much every other box, bag, jar, or can on the grocery store shelves. All of which, appearing extra tasty.

You wouldn't eat the "play food" in the kids' fake food packages, would you? Then why are we convinced that these factory-made foods are safe for human consumption? They share many of the same ingredients. We could do an entire book on the misleading's from our food industry, government agencies, and nutrition labels and a few people already have. For now, getting back on the topic of sugar I would like to introduce you to the devil in disguise. More than 50 different disguises you can find on nutrition labels. Such as...

The undercover criminal

Glucose, dextrose, fructose/fruit sugar, galactose, lactose, maltose, sucrose, levulose, sucralose, Splenda, beet sugar, brown sugar, cane juice crystals, cane sugar, castor sugar, coconut sugar, confectioners or powdered sugar, corn syrup solids, crystalline fructose, date sugar, demerara sugar, dextrin, diastatic malt. ethyl maltol, Florida crystals, golden sugar, glucose syrup solids, grape sugar, icing sugar, maltodextrin, muscovado sugar, panela sugar, raw sugar, sucanat, turbinado sugar, yellow sugar, agave nectar/syrup, barley malt, blackstrap molasses, brown rice syrup, buttered sugar/buttercream, caramel, carob syrup, corn syrup, evaporated cane juice, fruit juice, fruit juice concentrate, golden syrup, high Fructose Corn Syrup, honey, invert Sugar, malt syrup, maple syrup, molasses, rice syrup, refiners syrup, sorghum syrup, ethanol, brown rice sugar.

The side effects of excess sugar consumption generally start with some sort of inflammation, for me that inflammation was acne. The face was the start, then the back, chest, and shoulders. When the inflammation would go full blue flame I would have massive mountains on my neck, armpits and sometimes groin. I now know that excess processed sugar was the main culprit, and that the lymph system needs some help (the neck, pits, and groin areas are highways for your lymph system and mine was apparently malfunctioning). When I finally made the connection between the reaction and the cause I made the changes necessary. Sugar is highly addictive, and the journey has taken many years. I personally limit processed sugars to special occasions like birthdays and holidays. I don't go hog wild at these events because I know the consequence. After learning how to exercise correctly, eat properly, use hot/cold contrast therapy, and assist my lymph system through movement, dry brushing, and light massage I have smashed a lifelong issue with inflammation. Whole fruits fermented and/or sprouted seeds and grains in small amounts don't seem to have the same effect on me. Dairy on the other hand has this effect on both Kaitlyn and me. Even the glorified A2 milks and goat milks, raw and all, we have tried them.

Since humans express a wide variety of biochemical individuality, inflammation can be observed and felt in a multitude of ways. Including many auto-immune diseases. A beginning stage of glucose intolerance and sugar sensitivity leading to auto-immune diseases and inflammation normally begins with insulin resistance. When we consume sugars, especially sucrose and glucose the effects are more problematic. Our body must begin breaking it down immediately after consumption. The pancreas releases insulin into the blood to deal with those blood sugar levels without delay. If the pancreas does not produce the insulin, or not enough insulin, or even too much insulin, a diabetes diagnosis is around the corner. Insulin resistance left unresolved inevitably leads to diabetes.

The secretion of insulin is a normal and healthy reaction, the dose makes the poison. When you consume processed sugar all the time you have an abundance of insulin in your blood, which will eventually create a resistance to it, and that will lead to higher excretions, and more resistance until your pancreas can't keep up with the demand and eventually fails. Sometimes that dose isn't from just one binge meal, it's a chain of binge meals, days, weekends, weeks, months, years, decades, and/or passed down epigenetically. Remember, as our species evolved slowly over the last 2 million years, the availability of excessive amounts of sugar was extremely rare. One may have had the opportunity to sit beside a wild berry bush and indulge until the plant was empty but for liminal periods of the year, competing against birds, bears, other humans, and other berry lovers. And finding it at just the right time of ripeness.

A large modern apple has about 30gs of carbs/sugars while a wild crab apple has about 20gs. Humans have genetically modified the apple for size, sweetness (for palatability), longer seasons and larger yields. We have done the same type of modifying with basically every plant food that we eat today. And still, after about twenty thousand years of slow, purposeful genetic modification these plant foods provide nutritional value.

More than 34 million Americans have diabetes (about 1 in 10), and approximately 90-95% of them have type 2 diabetes. Type 2 diabetes most often develops in people over age 45, but more and more kids, teens and young adults are also developing it. (Quoted from the CDC) Type 2 diabetes is an impairment in the way the body regulates and uses sugar (glucose) as a fuel. This long-term (chronic) condition results in too much sugar circulating in the bloodstream. Eventually, high blood sugar levels can lead to disorders of the circulatory, nervous, and immune systems.

In type 2 diabetes, there are primarily two interrelated problems at work. Your pancreas does not produce enough insulin — a hormone that regulates the movement of sugar into your cells — and cells respond poorly to insulin and take in less sugar. (Mayo Clinic) Flip that food pyramid upside down because excess glucose (particularly processed) is not good for humans.

Type 1 diabetes is a chronic condition where little or no insulin production is observed due to an autoimmune reaction against the pancreas. Most observed symptoms include excessive thirst, frequent urination, sudden weight loss and weakness. Treatment includes lifestyle modifications and taking insulin to keep the sugar levels under control. (Focus Medica). Gestational diabetes of course is the one that some women experience during pregnancy where the symptoms and triggers are the same, but the condition is normally limited to the period during pregnancy.

Type 1 is the one you're born with, type 2 is the one that you create, starting with insulin sensitivity. Which, all humans experience at differing levels. Diabetes both 1 and 2 can lead to what many doctors have coined type 3 diabetes. Alzheimer's disease. Type III diabetes is the term to illustrate the relationship between type I, type II diabetes, and Alzheimer's disease. The progression from diabetes to Alzheimer's disease isn't entirely understood, but there are numerous links between the two diseases. The internal mechanism we discussed earlier; insulin resistance is a main risk factor, but they include metabolic risk factors such as hyper glycaemia. These risk factors are a result of inflammation.

Plants inhabited this planet long before anything larger than bacteria tried to eat them, they had adequate time to produce (through evolutionary trial and error, for both the plants and animals) substances that could make use of herbivores. Which didn't show up until about 300 million years ago, plants had roughly a 200-million-year head start on herbivores larger than bacteria. Highly addictive, useful, and not immediately life-threatening carbohydrates partnered with defense chemicals in plants ensured that their "predators" would not eat them entirely, but instead, spread their seeds, pollinate them, protect, and eventually dedicate millions of acres to harvest them where they would otherwise not be able to proliferate successfully on their own. Many plants have essentially and effectively turned animals into their custodians. This is obvious when we account for the fact that thousands of plants that do not use animals in their reproduction cycle are mostly toxic to eat, touch or even breath around. Such plants want nothing to do with animal disturbance, whilst their evolutionary counterparts want to manipulate us.

As Paul Saladino MD and author of "Carnivore Code" often says in slightly different ways, plants can't run away from predators, but they still have the same will to survive as an animal that can flee, hide, and fight predators so plants use special defense mechanisms like toxins. These toxins will slowly cause oxidative stress that will affect your health.

Poof! Uh... there goes your health

PUFA's, polyunsaturated fats. Saturated fats resist oxidation in the body and during cooking while PUFA's are easily oxidizable. Seed oils are a primary driver of oxidative stress in the western world when consumed in excess. PUFA's will undergo uncontrolled, spontaneous, non-digestive, anon non-enzymatic oxidative attacks while inside you. The body can handle some of the oxidative attacks using enzymes like catalase and compounds like glutathione but when the attacks are all day, every day, they exceed the limitations of the body causing high levels of inflammation and in turn upsetting homeostasis and this can lead to disease. Excess seed oil consumption leads to an increased dependence on sugars for energy, since inflammation is increased already the added sugars aren't coming to the rescue, they are coming to join in on the attack. Glen D Lawrence department of chemistry and biochemistry, Long Island University states that "PUFAs are important for production of a wide range of bioactive substances in the body, but like some vitamins and essential minerals, may become toxic when consumed in excess." For more information regarding seed oils, their lack of nutrition and surplus of negative side-effects read Dr. Cate Shanahan's book "Deep Nutrition".

Protect yourself and your family by learning to read and understand nutrition labels, and ingredient lists on packaged food items. From this point forward you shouldn't be purchasing many items that are packaged but for the ones that you do, be sure to read the labels. What's on the front of the package isn't always truthful. It's more of a billboard or a sales pitch. To know what's really in the item you'll have to dissect the label. For example, just the other day I picked up a bottle that read "Organic Olive Oil" in large lettering on the front, amongst other things that I did not thoroughly read. It was in a nice, dark green glass bottle and was priced as high as a *good* organic olive oil typically is. When we got to the checkout line Kaitlyn happened to see it and realizing that this was a brand we had not bought before she curiously inspected the label. What I had believed to be a glass of 100% organic olive oil was truthfully a mix of sunflower oil, canola oil, soybean oil, and olive oil. Granted, they were organic. This is why it's important to look beyond the flashy ads on the front and investigate the ingredients.

Nutrition labels are helpful, they tell you what is in your food, but they aren't entirely factual either. For example, a "serving" of canola oil may have ½ a gram of trans fat (fat that causes oxidative stress leading to cellular and DNA damage) but since it doesn't exceed ½ a gram per serving the label can read zero trans-fat, they can even advertise that it has zero trans-fat. Who only uses 1 tablespoon of canola oil though? Look in any restaurant kitchen and you'll find jugs upon jugs of cheap canola oil and find pots, pans, fryers, and skillets soaked in it. Cups and cups of it. There are 16 tablespoons in 1 cup. A typical fryer has anywhere from 3-6 cups. That's anywhere from 48 to 96 tablespoons, or 48-96 servings. Sure, you won't be drinking all this oil, at least I hope not. But this oil is soaking into your food and being re-heated for days or even weeks and becoming more rancid and toxic each time. Yet, they can say there are no trans-fats.

The popular and poisonous French fry that Americans enjoy so much are soaking in anywhere from 24 to 48 grams of trans fat and you don't need to know it. At least that's how the FDA appears to feel. About 25% worth of the weight in French fries are oils that soaked in from the frying process. The average American consumes 16 pounds of French fries per year, That's about four pounds or eight and a half cups of hydrogenated oil per year. 136 servings or 68 grams of trans fat. That's from French fries alone, this doesn't include the rest of the meal or any other meal for that matter. The American Heart Association recommends less than 1% of your diet should contain trans-fat. Imagine what other foods you eat on a regular basis that could be soaked in trans-fat. The average American is consuming way more than 1%. How can anyone expect to represent the best version of themselves when their body is constantly fighting off internal, oxidative stress? (Ditch all oils besides fruit oils like coconut, olive oil and avocado oil, they are much better than seed oils but animal fats like tallow, lard, ghee, and grass-fed butter appear to be the best in my research.)

Eliminating or limiting your processed sugar and vegetable oil intake will immediately elevate your health and attitude. Subsequently improving your wealth and karma as you re-introduce yourself to nature and the circle of life. The value of your life will increase tremendously. No one said that it would be easy, but it's worth it. I have been working on the road for over a decade and understand the gas station, middle of nowhere grocery store struggle, I know the extreme fatigue state when ghrelin levels are through the roof and all you can think of is eating something horrible. I've been there. It's not always an easy road to tote when raising a family in the modern world either. But it is worth it. Learn to meal prep it could be a literal life saver.

CHAPTER THREE

PREGNANCY NUTRITION, FITNESS, WELLNESS, AND ANCESTRAL LIVING FOR MAMA (KAITLYN SWEET)

When I was younger, up until my early twenty's nutrition was not a word I ever used. I was naturally on the smaller side with my body weight and could eat nothing but junk food without gaining weight. But looking back on my life there were SO MANY signs that I was unhealthy.

I had acne, I was constantly fatigued, and emotional often but the part that led me to holistic nutrition and eventually to energy healing was wanting to become a mom. I was not regular with my menstrual cycle for years; in fact, it was common for me to just get 1 or 2 periods a year. After my first couple random periods, my mom took me to the OBGYN for insight on my cycle and what we could do to get on a consistent cycle and help the pain. When I did get a period, I would have a tremendous amount of pain & cramps with the menstrual cycle, bad body aches, belly aches, head aches you name it! I thought this was okay because every girl I knew that had periods experienced cramps, so I thought it was "normal", even though mine were excruciating.

After running a few different tests and blood work they found nothing to be terribly wrong, but they did inform my mom that later in life it would be very difficult for me to become pregnant, it had something to do with hormonal imbalances (probably from my junk food habits), looking back this seems like something was truly wrong, but I guess they didn't want to alarm us. At the time, they wanted to put me on a type of birth control that would "help" my ovulation time and hormones. My mom thought I was much too young to be on birth control (13yrs old) so she opted out and said my body would figure it out in time. Now, I understand the time and place for medicine, but I also deeply believe in a holistic approach and so did my mother. For that occasion, especially due to the large number of cases where women and their children deal with negative side-effects from birth-control medications it was a hard "no" from my mom.

We left and the years to follow I would still have crazy periods at random times. Finally, around the age of eighteen, I met my husband who was at the time a boyfriend and after months of dating I told him about what I had going on fertility wise. He said that he was also told that he had slim chances of having children because of a severe hernia when he was a small child.

After accepting this fact, it made us a bit closer and didn't really affect how we felt about each other, if anything it helped us feel more comfortable. No blame could be cast on either of us if we had trouble conceiving in the future. We also weren't ready to have children just yet but enjoyed our lives together & honestly the infrequent periods at this point in my life were almost convenient because I didn't have to deal with them, the excruciating and debilitating pain I felt during the periods made me never want one anyways.

When we first started trying for children, we were so young! I was 21 and Trenton was 24, we had been married for about a year. (Crazy I know, but when you know... you know). I had gone to the OBGYN for about a year trying to find out what was going on with me and if there was anything medically, I could do. We found out that there was nothing medically wrong, but of course, I could take a script and see if it helped. I chose to leave it in God's hands that October and never filled the script... late

November I was pregnant. This story is so deep for me because when you are in the trenches of something like this it is an indescribable feeling for you... watching others become pregnant and having little babies that you are DREAMING of having, when you are dreaming so hard for that reality for yourself and your marriage. Realistically, we had been having completely unsafe sex for like three years by this time, we just didn't put the word "trying" on it before that first of marriage.

Before I got pregnant Trenton and I had made a commitment to clean up our lifestyle a little and try to get into better shape. Trenton knew all the ways to exercise from playing minor-league football and being an athlete prior, but we knew nothing about eating correctly. We both still believed at this point that processed carbs like pasta were good for you. We did make some changes though, we cut the alcoholic drinks when we went out to eat, along with the appetizers and desserts. Started walking more often and spending more time outdoors, we got gym memberships and started working out. We did the best we could with what we knew at this point in our lives. With these minor changes I believe God blessed us with my first pregnancy.

When we found out I was pregnant I immediately started researching how I could have a healthy pregnancy, for the sake of my baby, but also first-time moms know we fear gaining weight and stretch marks! I was so scared that I wouldn't see my pre-pregnancy body ever again & every mom out there including the ones in my family assured me that I could toss my size 1's & 0's in the trash because I would never see that waistline again. This FREAKED me out! I stopped the consumption of any type of "fast food" or "pop" at this point I for sure knew that wasn't good for me or the little babe, but prior to this I ate in a drive-thru at least twice a weeks & always got loaded down sugary sweet tea & flurry. This honestly

99

was my biggest step into the right direction but the hardest one for me. Old habits die HARD. I would literally dream of these foods in my sleep & smell them out of the air when we passed these fast-food joints especially with pregnancy cravings. Looking back, I can see how deep the addiction of this food was for me.

I gained quite a bit of weight despite this change during my first pregnancy, about 50 lbs. I thought that was good, since everyone was telling me I was going to gain a ton of weight. This extra fifty pounds was the weight gain after birth. Everyone says that it is perfectly fine and "normal" to gain this amount of weight, but I wasn't happy with it. I did what I knew to do, I ate plenty of servings of fruit, vegetables, & meat. I made smoothies, took a prenatal, ate when I was hungry, also with the mind set of eating for two & kind of gave into cravings of my famous ice cream joint at least twice a week. I also consumed a ton of carbs, processed ones. I did what I thought was right. We had our amazing, beautiful first baby girl perfect in health & weight and that's all you could EVER pray for as a parent. Ultimately, as parents we do what we believe is the best thing for our kiddos through our hearts and with every ounce of love inside of us.

Very shortly after giving birth to our daughter Trenton knocked me up again! About 7 weeks after giving birth! We did not use any protection because, well it took us that long to get pregnant the first time and I was told if I was breast feeding, I was unable to have another. That is obviously not true, or the minor changes had made us super fertile. We had two beautiful babies 11 months apart, and it worked out to be the most incredible thing that could have happened to us. I remember when our second was born our sweet nurse said to me while looking over our baby on the table in the delivery room "If this baby scored any higher on the newborn screening test, I would believe his name would be Jesus." We laughed about this and beamed with love over our newborn. There was so much worry with these pregnancies being so close because of the risk of the body not fully healing. My experience was a really good one, but I believe this had a lot to do with the lifestyle changes we were being called to make at this time as well as the education we were being lead to. I was in school online during this pregnancy earning my holistic nutrition certification which took about 10 months as well as working part time in a salon. I felt so naturally called in the direction of health it was odd for me! I could not explain why I felt the need to be in that route other than saying it was for my babies & superficial reasons. But looking back I was and am so passionate about the topic of healing the body. The feeling I have on this topic just ignites an inner fire that grows as I feed it.

With my second pregnancy I only gained about thirty-five pounds. We ate so much better because I had a better understanding of what nutrition was. I was completing my studies to become a Holistic Nutritionist at the end of this pregnancy and working towards applying other healing strategies to my body.

The years to follow I deeply studied nutrition and exercise and how it works in and around the body. I became primarily plant-based with the consumption of meat MAYBE once every two weeks. I had studied and learned so much against dairy, meat & fat and honestly felt good with this diet change because it was so much better than my previous years of chips, cake, pasta, alcohol, & pop. I also did a very strict calorie count diet around 1200 a day while excessively working out 2 hours a day (a lot of body weight training & walking). The only time I looked at a nutrition label was to see how many calories were in something. I would survive on primarily fruits, veggies, random low-calorie bars, and low-cal ice cream's if my calorie count was low enough. I looked at calories like currency. I only drank black coffee, teas that helped lose weight like green, rooibos, and oolong teas. I also ate quick "healthy" meals from the freezer section that you could pop in the microwave with maybe 220 calories. This did help me drop weight down to about 120lbs within 3 months. Because of how dramatically improved this diet was compared to my previous one, I was feeling better, but after a few months I noticed some changes that started to present to me the shortcomings of a diet void of healthy meat.

Flash way forward to about a year before I became pregnant with our 3rd little babe, (about 3 years since our first daughter was born) I was in the best shape of my life at that point. I worked out about 6 days a week with weights and HIIT cardio and was still eating primarily plant based. I saw amazing results and had a good amount of energy, but I would have these crashes a few times a day where my energy was so low that I needed to nap. I would get easily frustrated and annoyed, seemingly out of nowhere. This would lead me to consume more carbs and then I would feel back at my game... & then crash yet again. I thought maybe I was just super busy (which I was) but not that busy. I had lost all the body weight I ever wanted to and gained a good amount of muscle in the process; I had the start of a four pack, but it never progressed beyond that. My husband was learning a ton about nose to tail, animal-based diets at this time and not that I was vegan, but I didn't agree with the idea of eating meat multiple times a week let alone multiple times a day... For me, it wasn't about the yogi idea of bad karma from eating animals or the idea that humans didn't evolve eating animals, it was honestly because everything I learned in my holistic nutrition classes was based on the premise that meat caused disease, cancer & pre-mature aging.

102

We would get into large conversations about both of our sides, both making sense and having good arguments and data to support them, but we never really saw eye to eye.

Not only was I unsure of eating meat multiple times a day I was even fearful of adding dairy. I have always known that I have crazy reactions to dairy & processed sugar, but I thought it was normal. I had horrible body acne as a teenager because of it. Dairy would break me out within hours of consuming it, no matter the kind and the effects would last for days. Dairy might really work for some people and if it is raw, organic, 100% grass-fed, regeneratively farmed I think you should keep it a part of your diet but for me, and Trenton alike, dairy is a no-go.

I learned so much in my 3rd pregnancy about being pregnant, things that I wish were taught to me prior. But I am grateful for the ability to learn and teach what I have learned. I bought books on books on books, when I was very early in my first trimester because I wanted to fully understand the pregnant body. I mean it's so different, a woman even grows a new organ (the placenta) to supply for the baby! I was so thirsty to know how a baby developed and how my body created life. My first motive was, I was going to attend a 200hr YTT (yoga teacher training) course in the fall where I would be starting at 34 weeks pregnant (so crazy) and giving birth in the very beginning of it and attending Reiki & YTT training 3 days later after giving birth with my newborn, breast feeding her in class. (Story for another time). Also running my clothing store and taking care of our other two babes & working out as hard as my body would allow & doing low temp sauna sessions (<110*) while my husband worked an insane schedule... I needed all the true nutrition I could get especially because I was having these crashes! I knew I could not continue like this, and I felt like my progress had really tapered off.

I delved deeply into two books that taught me a ton, and… of course I learned that Trenton was right about a lot of nose-to-tail nutrition he was researching as well. I dove deep into the books "Real food for pregnancy" & "The first forty days." I wanted a true, natural, and comfortable pregnancy and post-partum experience. Not one where I rushed and felt rushed in my healing processes and push my body to recover and work out asap. I wanted to do it like our ancestors did. Peacefully, nutritionally, with the health of me and baby the number one priority. Healing and growing simultaneously in the same space. The previous experiences were insane, to say the least. Trenton had minimal time off work and he had to fight with his employers (literally) to stay off for as long as he did. This time Trenton took off a total of 4 weeks, 2 weeks prior to giving birth and two weeks after birth. We both wanted him to take more time off, but we needed the income.

I didn't want to have post-partum anxiety… which I did the first two pregnancy's because I believe I never healed right; it was so rushed. No one's fault, just the way our society is. As soon as a woman gives birth she is asked when she plans to return to work. Like, give me some time to heal and enjoy my baby! The pressure to get back to work and back "into shape" is so strong, and from so many angles, but specifically internally for me. I wasn't kind to myself, I was so anxious to get back to "me" that I didn't care the state I was in "now", the internal cultural drive and the outside pressure made me rush back to my duties outside of being a mother.

This is what I learned, during pregnancy you need a tremendous amount of minerals, fat, protein (amino acids), water, and vitamins from herbs, organ meats, fresh meats, & fermented foods. This also goes for post-partum which we forget about! I adored my post-partum experience every time … those sweet two days after giving birth are my favorite! My Third time giving birth was the calmest, sweetest post-partum experience I have had. Yes, you are still in pain, very tired & yes you are still riding an emotional roller coaster but not to the point of where I was in previous birth stories. This was SO MUCH DIFFERENT, I listened to my body in a different light. I also combined reiki energy healing post-partum and end of pregnancy. Post-partum health is very particular in health as well, a woman needs certain foods for good energy in and around the body, easy consumables all at warm temperatures, no processed sugars, very limited fruits if any postpartum first 2 weeks. Healing herbs for baths and belly wraps for your muscles, to lay in positions that are best for healing your body, mindfulness and deep healing liquids that contain immense amounts of minerals for your body. It's just as important as creating the baby to help heal the body after it gives birth to its beautiful creation with the help of God. When you are pregnant you are in a flowing state of "chi" when you are giving birth there is a significant amount of blood loss which puts your body into a "yin" state(cold). During this first month you do NOT consume cold items only hot items and mostly liquids. You want to eat foods that are easily digested and high in bioavailable forms of minerals, vitamins, and nutrients. This is so important and to make it easier I made a ton of meal prepped bone broths, electrolyte drinks (harmonized water, trace minerals, lemon, ginger, pink salt) while pregnant in mason jars so Trenton or I could grab them out of the freezer for me later. I also have an amazing recipe for a home-made coconut milk egg nog that Trenton made for me post-partum!

Examples of foods not to eat until at least two weeks post-partum are cold foods & drinks, ice cream, bananas, watermelon, soy, cold smoothies, any fruit other than goji berries, red dates & very small amounts of berries (this was hard for me). I learned instead to consume foods that were truly nutritious, and bioavailable (meaning that the body must do very little to the nutrients to use them, efficiency is always better). The books I mentioned earlier were loaded with recipes for post-partum and to my surprise they were animal based. In Chinese medicine, Celtic origins, eastern countries, and Native American origins they had all been eating this way for many generations prioritizing warm nutritious animal-based meals for women that were pregnant and post-partum. Warm bone broths & marrow soups, liver, heart, kidney, cooked greens, cooked ginger, meats of all kinds, cognees, pickled & fermented warm items & oddly enough no pure water... this was shocking. I found that post-partum every tiny bit of nutrients matter. If you had a liquid, water could be the base, like tea or broth of some sort, just no plain water. Pure water actually isn't that great for anyone, what you are drinking should nourish you, not take away your nourishment. Pure water desperately wants minerals to replenish it, essentially your water wants to be hydrated. So, if your water is plain and has no minerals in it, it's going to take them from your body. Vice-versa, if your water has extra minerals in it, then your body is going to keep its minerals and absorb some from the water.

During this pregnancy I converted over to only consuming organic fruits and vegetables if this is not in your budget, go for organic frozen, it is much cheaper than fresh! If that's still too expensive, I get it, conventional fruit washed off is better than no fruit. I consumed organs from animals at least twice a week typically liver (this was so hard at first) there was a ton of research I found on its benefits, numerous documentaries, podcasts, books etc. My husband and I made a ton of loaded down mineral bone broths and froze them in the freezer for after-birth quick meals. I consumed salmon, bison, elk, boar, beef, lamb just flat out a wide range of meat while pregnant. I also started cooking with fats other than coconut oil like tallow, olive oil on low temps you can also do

106

grass-fed ghee & grass-fed butters. Dairy doesn't treat me well but if it works for you then great!

Carbs are super debatable while pregnant I'm going to touch on this very lightly with the knowledge that helped me dive deeper for what I needed for my body. I was told carb intake should be 45-65% of your diet (250-420 grams) of a 2,000 calories per day diet. Diet of 2,200-2,600 while pregnant for a person *requiring* 2,000 calories per day. This high of a carb intake has been observed to cause obesity in utero though. Despite the copious amounts of carbs pushed on pregnant women in the U.S. most cultures around the world consume far less amounts, in 2011 a study on hunter and gatherers from around the world, 229 women in modern hunter gatherer groups consumed an average of 16-22% of their calories from carbohydrates. Women in colder climates consumed far less carbohydrates 3-15% compared to the women near the equator who consumed 29-34% carbohydrates because of living in a hunter gatherer community they ate what was abundant that's why warmer climates ate higher carbs because of the fruit abundance. Even with the abundant of fruit in the area they still rarely exceeded 30% carbs in their diet. Yet, our government is teaching us that we need 45-65%?!

Being pregnant in todays' world means that you are going to experience a lot of things, things that ancestral women most likely did not. One thing is for sure, despite your efforts to be a strong, healthy woman you are going to experience cravings. An evolutionary trait designed to ensure momma and baby are receiving adequate nutrition. Early ancestral women carrying babies would have been given an abundance of nutritious food from the tribe. A pregnant woman was protected and prized by her people, populations were low, and *every single child and birthing mother* was a blessing, they did everything they could to protect her and make sure her and baby were healthy. Nutritional intake for a pregnant momma is important for both her and the babe. So, snacking was important, and strong cravings for a variety of foods, (originally correlating with highly nutritious and caloric foods) this trait now leads most women straight to the ice-cream shop.

Don't fight the cravings, don't indulge in cheesecake either, also don't feel guilt for wanting those things. Here are some examples of low carb snacks during pregnancy that will help stave off the sugary indulgences and allow you to remain as healthy as can be.

Use a wide variety of nuts and seeds, like lentils, beans, and chia. Sprout your seeds beforehand by soaking them in a liquid, this is very important because of the amount of plant toxins in them, sprouting breaks them down significantly and makes them healthier. I love to make a chia pudding with chia seeds, full fat coconut milk &, raw honey this fills you up with dense nutrition while giving you that *something sweet*. I also make avocado pudding; this one is going to satisfy every chocolate pudding craving you have ever had. It took years of me perfecting something so simple. Avocado pudding is avocados, coconut milk, cacao & raw organic honey. THAT'S IT. I sometimes add nutmeg or pink salt to a batch or get more adventurous with other flavors. I also love to have dark chocolate in the cabinet, ALWAYS look at the ingredients. I've found a great brand that make their chocolate with coconut sugar, cacao, cacao butter & pink salt. Small amounts of plain Greek yogurt with berries if dairy serves you well, dates, figs, avocado's, sweet bell peppers, fresh celery, eggs boiled or deviled, olives, dill pickles, pesto, cherry tomatoes, pine nuts, goat cheese, sheep cheese, meat, cauliflower, coconut milk, salmon, bacon, Grass fed beef, dark chocolate that is (75% cacao or more no refined sugar, look for coconut sugar or maple syrup & honey as sweetener).

Stay away from fruit juices. An 8oz glass of orange juice has 30g sugar, equivalent to an 8 oz pop. Yes, this is by far a better choice than pop but still high in natural sugars & your body responds almost identically and has the same blood sugar spike when consumed (explains all the crashes on fruit I was having). Infused waters are a great choice like cucumber & lime, peach & basil, strawberry & kiwi, coconut water, Kombuchas, teas, coffee (no more than 16 oz daily, go for decaf while pregnant), green smoothies & my favorite ever mitochondria enhancing drink, Hot Cacao with unsweetened coconut milk, cacao butter & unsweetened cacao powder. I've honestly made it a mission especially in pregnancy to find ways to satisfy my sweet tooth without it being dangerous to my body. I've got quite a stack of recipes that I have come up with for this!

Prioritize highly nutritious animal protein while pregnant minimum 1 gram of protein per pound that you weigh while pregnant. Slow cooked meats are your BFF here, and variety is key. Eat lamb, beef, bison, venison, elk, duck, chicken, salmon, trout etc. Make sure that the birds are pasture raised and organic, ruminant species pasture raised, 100% grass fed, organic, for seafood always choose wild-caught, for fish always choose small breeds, check for color added through feed on the back of the fish package (you don't want that in your body), organ meats from all animals, bone broth or stocks, eggs, sprouted seeds beans & legumes, nuts (variety). This ensures a great balance in amino acids and other key vitamins & minerals. Seafood & salmon are great sources of Omega 3s. Red meat is very high in iron especially organ meats, you need lots of iron. Slow cooked meats and bone broths contain glycine in high amounts. Liver and kidney contain up to two hundred times the levels of vitamin b12 than muscle meats.

Try to always go for grass fed & finished it contains much higher levels of beta carotene, vitamin E and omega threes.

Bring your mind to your plate before eating, check in with your body for 30 seconds before you start eating and take in a few deep breaths, so you are not stressfully eating. Be mindful of your meal or snack and don't rush to get through it. (Easier said than done with kiddos I know but it's important, make every moment of your life worth it.) I love the topic of child birth & nutrition for baby, mama, daddy & toddlers!

Working out while pregnant

Exercising while pregnant is a topic that a lot of people go back and forth on, but it is completely safe to exercise while carrying your little one. In fact, The American Congress of Obstetricians and Gynecologists suggests in there guidelines to engage in at least 30 minutes a day of moderate exercise everyday of the week while pregnant as long as you do not have a serious health condition. I however did moderate exercise while pregnant with my second child but did not do any type of exercise with my first child besides working full time as a hair stylist my entire pregnancy. Come my third pregnancy I was fully engaged in exercise, yoga, barre & strength training. I did carry this on throughout my third pregnancy with adjusting as my belly grew and my body was changing. I did inversions, head stands and HIIT cardio up until the middle of my second trimester, I was around 27 weeks pregnant when I decided to change up certain activities. Keynote is I listened to my body; I did what was right for me in body each day & each week.

When I first found out I was pregnant with my third baby some exercises in my lower abdominal where not fun to do, I remember around 12 weeks feeling a weird tension in my lower abdominal wall when I would do any type of ab work, but this only lasted for about a week. Once I felt okay to pick up light core work again, I did until my bump started getting bigger. Engaging the appropriate muscles in an abdominal work out while earlier in pregnancy will decrease your chances of developing diastasis recti. During pregnancy, the abdominal wall is gapped to accommodate the growing baby because the linea alba (connective tissue that connects both sides of the *six pack*) must stretch for the babe. It is super common to have some degree of diastasis recti in the third trimester of pregnancy at least 67% of women do. Women who work out during pregnancy have a much lower chance of developing this long term and have quicker healing time post-partum, if you choose not to work out while pregnant you have a higher risk of developing diastasis recti. In another study women who were inactive during pregnancy had a 90% incidence of diastasis recti compared to only 12.5% among active women who performed the correct core exercises.

A great exercise to do while pregnant that you can do while sitting is transversus abdominis muscle activation. This will create a muscular brace around your mid-section so that rectus abdominus is not taking the grunt of all the work. When you engage the "corset muscles" by gently drawing in your naval towards your spine & up towards your rib cage you are engaging these muscles. You can also do this through light breath work.

Its also important to strengthen the pelvic floor while pregnant to keep proper alignment of the torso, think about it... you are about to engage in the craziest experience of your life, giving birth to a baby! You want to give your body all the tools it will need to be ready for this and to recover from such an incredible, divine experience and you want to experience this at your full potential. With all the tools in your toolbox in your head you can just pull them out and put them to work, how empowering is that?! We should train and prepare our bodies for childbirth, it's the greatest physical task our bodies will take on; why would we not prepare mentally, physically, emotionally & nutritionally for this. I feel like so often that exercise during pregnancy is overlooked, we are beautiful human beings creating life on this earth bringing love to an unborn child we need to be in tip-top condition and should take the time to be there for our bodies while in this process. Of course, you should relax but you should also do what your body needs and listen to its needs that come from its energy field and your heart.

Moves you should avoid especially when the bump is getting bigger in the end of the second trimester are crunches, roll ups, plank, side body crunches, toe touches, bicycles anything that is bulging your midline during exercises. Pay super close attention to what abdominal muscles you are engaging, you want to be engaging your transverse abdominal muscles by bracing your abdominal muscles before exertion. MODIFY YOUR EXERCISES.

Working out my entire third pregnancy up until my due date was hard, I modified a ton of exercises to fit where my body was each day. Towards the end of my third trimester, I did mostly yoga and was becoming certified in YTT (yoga teacher training) this helped so much with giving birth and pregnancy aches and pains. I never had swelling in my feet or hands like other pregnancies I genuinely believe it was because of my yoga practices that I applied while pregnant!

My favorite yoga moves that are fantastic for mom and bump in third trimester are cat & cow stretches, child's pose, rag doll, downward dog, mountain pose, half pigeon, happy baby, tree pose, figure four, warrior two, side angle pose, camel pose, and any type of hip opener I CRAVED. As the bump grows you will find spinal twists and full body twists are hard and do not feel so great on the bump or uterus at least for me I stopped when the crunchy feeling started.

The first and second trimester you can pretty much keep up with your same routine as always and just watch how your body feels in each position as you flow and the bump gets bigger, obviously any belly down exercises in yoga or training should be completely avoided & trust me you will be surprised how many there truly are! I totally didn't realize how many moves where belly down till I was in class and had to switch it up. Don't over stretch, its super easy to do while pregnant for one it feels amazing to get deep into those hips and butt muscles to release tension from the bump and hip shifting, two your body is producing high amounts of the hormone relaxin, as the name implies relaxes your ligaments while your body shifts and moves. Without relaxin, your body wouldn't be able to stretch the way it does to give birth to your beautiful baby! Use caution when getting deeper in your stretches judge by how far you would typically go and don't go much further past that (even if it does feel amazing) because you are doing more damage than good if the ligament is overstretched, or a muscle is pulled especially in that third trimester when your babe is bigger and you have more weight in your mid-section. During your pregnancy, exercise alignment is important, so good posture and correct footing while exercising is key. As your center of gravity shifts and your body starts to grow you need to watch your stance. Try and make sure your hips are not too far forward or tucking in your tailbone to counterbalance the bump. Instead of leaning forward and letting the baby pull you forward imagine your body growing taller and taller this will naturally center your gravity and spine. Think about perfect alignment in your body, roll your shoulders back, shoulders over ribs, ribs over hips, hips over knees and even weight in all four corners of your feet. I honestly just picture a steel beam in my head to create strength and balance in my body. This helps me feel strong and keep alignment during my practice & when I am doing balance work. Now, get moving!

Meditation While Pregnant

I love to meditate especially while pregnant, this gives at least five minutes of my day to be with just myself and my bump. I feel like the best advice I can give on this topic is just let the thoughts flow by, observe them with out an emotional attachment and then just let them go and focus on your breath. Slowly let each muscle in your body relax, melt into your space. Ground down through your pelvic floor and think of your connection to mother earth. Slowly focusing on each chakra point as you move up the body from the root, sacral, solar plexus, heart, throat, third eye and your crown.

During meditation think about the joy, love, and gratitude you have for the experience of creating your child, the opportunity your body has to create and the connection and love you feel for your baby. This helped me when I felt anxious about supplying for our little one or having everything we needed, it also helped whenever I would feel overwhelmed or sad by a situation, to be brought back to this beautiful purpose my body has and had in that moment. Meditation is your own experience and how your body feels; there is no right or wrong way of doing it, just go with the flow of stillness and breath and it will lead you.

Making meditation a daily practice should be something you strive for at all stages of your life, pregnant, menstruating, or just plain living life. Meditation isn't always sitting cross-legged on a special pillow with your hands in mudra, chanting "Ommm", listening to bells, with patchouli burning all around you, but... that is also pretty awesome. You can meditate in many ways, just sitting still, watching the birds while drinking our morning coffee and just focusing on them, not on lifes mysteries and problems. You can meditate while walking the dog, focusing on the sounds you hear, the scents you smell around you, or your breath. You can meditate any time, anywhere. But, for the sake of maintaining your sanity as a momma, I highly suggest carving out at least thirty minutes a day where you can be alone, in a safe and quiet place with no disturbances and meditate.

Breathwork While pregnant

Breath work while pregnant should be kept light and easy, nothing crazy or super long breath holds. An example would be box breathing which is 4 seconds inhale, 4 seconds of holding the breath, 4 seconds of exhale, 4 seconds hold, repeat this for 1 to 2 minutes. If you ever feel lightheaded or like you will pass out during breath work stop and take a break; relax you do not need to stress your body, but light breath work should be fine and healthy for you during pregnancy. Another breathing exercise I did my entire pregnancy was simply observing my breath during meditation. I would see how much breath came in and out on a normal breathing cycle. If your breath in is longer than your breath out, you are anxious if your breath out is longer than your breath in this could mean you are giving too much of your energy away. Try and balance your breath equally in as out, if you are purposefully looking to calm the body take a 5 second breath in and a 7 second breath out, this will change the bodies response into a relaxed state when purposefully done. Breath of fire should be skipped in second & third trimester (also skipped when menstruating) and ujjayi breath can be practiced throughout pregnancy as long as it feels right in your body.

Breathing is one of the most difficult things to focus on, it's so boring. Which is why they say that if you can focus on your breath for a selected amount of time, you can focus on anything, any time. You take roughly 22,000 breaths per day, I think that focusing on a couple hundred of them per day is an easy ask. Especially knowing that breathwork alone has been shown to dramatically reduce the risk of disease and has even played roles in miraculous events where disease or cancer was beaten.

Mudras, a breathwork tool

Mudras are a sacred symbolic gesture you do in yoga or meditation practices. They are ways to channel your vital flow and energy source "prana." By doing different hand mudras you can source different energy flows, elements, or meridians in the hands. There is the gesture of knowledge "Gyan Mudra" which is tip of thumb to index finger while the other three fingers are free. The gesture of the earth "Prithvi Mudra" gently touch the tip of the ring finger and thumb while the other three fingers are stretched free. The gesture of life "Prana Mudra" ring finger and pink finger to tip of thumb gently keep other two finger stretched. The fire hand gesture "Suraya Mudra" fold the ring finger and touch the tip at the base of the thumb, while the tip of the thumb presses into the second phalax bone on the ring finger. The gesture of water "Varun Mudra" slightly touch the tip of the thumb with the little finger (pinky finger) the rest of the fingers should be unstressed and let freely. The gesture of air "Vayu Mudra" fold the index finger and press the second phalax bone with tip of thumb and tip of index finger should touch the base of the thumb. Those are the five basic mudras you can use! I love playing around with each mudra in different styles of yoga and meditation, they help with different moods and pains you may be having in the body or mind. They are an awesome tool to use even when driving in the car or giving childbirth (at the beginning when the pain is more manageable, breath work is so good for managing pain during childbirth!)

CHAPTER FOUR

EMF'S THE GOOD , THE BAD, AND THE WTF

We can't see them, we can't touch, smell, or taste them. But we are surrounded by them constantly and at the cellular level, every single one of them is received and interpreted. They exist both naturally and unnaturally. Biological organisms have their own, the planet itself has one, the sun, your smart phone, the wiring in your home, even pipes with city water flowing through them have one. At certain frequencies they are beneficial for biological systems and at other frequencies they are deadly. What has been coined "extremely low frequencies" have been seen to cause twice the occurrence of leukemia in children. Parts of the spectrum above extremely low and below the highest frequency known as gamma rays like infrared are known to be beneficial and even necessary for human life. What are we talking about here and what makes one frequency deadly and another healthy?

"Everything is energy and that's all there is to it." Albert Einstein. At the quantum level (the smallest known level of existence) everything vibrates. At the atomic level every*thing* vibrates at a specific frequency. Contact by differing frequencies can disrupt, influence, and/or alter another *things* frequency. The documentary "What the bleep do we know" discusses how music and sound waves (vibrations) literally change the molecular structure of water. The book "The Secret Life of Plants" by Peter

Tompkins and Christopher Bird discuss many ways that plants communicate and react to things at a vibrational level. Like growing towards a rock with beneficial minerals in it, and away from an identical looking rock with harmful chemicals. Also growing towards pleasant or happy music and growing away from mad and sad music. Our entire world communicates and responds to vibrations and frequencies on a moment-to-moment basis. "If you want to find the secrets to the Universe, think in terms of energy, frequency, and vibration." Nikola Tesla.

The book "The Intention Experiment" by Lynne McTaggart discusses in depth how just the frequency of intention changes the world around you. Good intentions and bad alike influence the world around us on a scientifically verifiable level. Emotions are energies in motion, that motion in the form of waves has a frequency that as it travels will influence and interact with the frequencies around it. When you can feel someone's vibe, you can tell that they are in a bad mood just by being around them, or when the rest of the crowd at a concert or game is hyped up and you can't help but be amped up to, these are examples of someone else's frequency affecting your own. It is important to remain in control of your energy so that other people's energy does not harmfully impact you.

There are many terms by which the spectrum that these frequencies travel in has been coined. The ether or luminiferous ether has been proven, then unproven now speculated as true but misunderstood again. The ether is the theoretical substance that acts as the medium for the transmission of electromagnetic frequencies and is believed to permeate all matter and space. This ether appears to exist everywhere and is constant, potentially controlled and maintained by the Higgs field or dark matter, no one has put an accepted scientific term on it yet.

Traversing through this space there are waves of every imaginable frequency, and more. Electro-magnetic frequencies travel through a substance that is still considered theoretical and exist in a state of matter that you may not even know exists. Speaking plainly, science doesn't have a lot of answers etched into stone when it comes to this topic.

We are taught the three states of matter, solid, liquid, and gas but they generally leave out plasma, the state in which nearly all matter in the universe exists as we just mentioned, EMFs are plasma. Earthly plasma examples are lightning, fire, neon signs, fluorescent lights, welding arcs, plasma TVs, auroras, and electricity. For the frequency surrounding one's physical body you may have heard terms like aura, biofield, or akasha. The depictions of halos are thought to be connected to one's field of energy as well. In civilizations around the world, you can find evidence of the people's knowledge of the biofield in their language, religion, and ceremonial practices. Many depictions of Saints, spiritual leaders, Gods, Goddesses, Shamans, High Priests, and the like are depicted with strong auras, halos and an overall abundance of light around their physical body in some way. Relating to what light-workers and spiritual leaders today know as energy centers or chakras. Eileen Day McKusick the author of "Electric Body, Electric Health" describes in her experience, aura's extending up to twelve feet away from a person's physical body but most commonly six feet. She uses tuning forks to scientifically verify this. Six to twelve feet is a lot of influence that you are both giving and receiving from the quantum world around you. Essentially, don't let external bullshit disturb your energy, and don't let your internal bullshit disturb others.

The history of EMFs

Up until about 100 years ago, the EMFs that our atoms lived amongst were natural. The ether soup of electro-magnetic plasmas that we resided in was coherent. Today, the plasma soup is very incoherent, constantly pulsing, and incomprehensible.

Frequencies are the number of waves that pass through a fixed point per second. Frequencies are measured in hertz, abbreviated Hz. EMFs come from natural and artificial sources. Natural EMFs like Lightning and sunlight possess benefits for health at the cellular level. Unless of course you're struck by said lightning bolt or in outer space without a radiation protecting suit or spacecraft protecting you from the suns powerful EMFs. Artificial ones like your microwave and the wiring in your home are known to disrupt the function of your cells. The higher the frequency the higher the risk, the longer the exposure at lower levels, the higher the risk. This is why your dentist puts a lead blanket over you when giving you an X-ray and then hides somewhere safe while the machine is on, X-rays are amongst the highest frequency waves and very short periods of exposure are known to cause irreversible biological damage.

There is a massive difference in frequencies between natural and artificial. Humanity evolved in direct contact with the Earth which has a natural electromagnetic frequency of 8.7 hertz, while the electromagnetic frequency radiated by our electric grid is between 50 and 60 hertz. That is almost seven times greater than the natural EMF we evolved in. The EMFs of microwaves and cell phones can be thousands of times greater than 50-60hz. Another difference between the frequencies is the pulse. Alternating currents pulse, and direct currents do not. The Earths electrical frequency and magnetic field are DC (direct current). While our entire electric grid is AC (alternating current). All batteries are DC. Our nervous systems synapsis and signals function like a battery sending electrons in one direction. The sodium: potassium pump in our cells is essentially a biological battery. Our bodies are designed to work with direct current not alternating current.

Nikola Tesla found that AC travels further distances than DC without losing voltage. Voltage is basically the *pressure* of electricity. Unfortunately for humans and unforeseen by Tesla, DC would have been a much better electrical system for the safety of biological organisms. Scientists have been going back in history and comparing heart attacks and mortality after learning that biological systems malfunction more often during variations in the magnetic fields during solar flares and magnetic storms. As they follow these cycles through history it has been identified that, definitively, biological systems are damaged and disrupted when variations of 20% or more from regular frequencies are observed. Yet our electrical grid was built on almost 700% variation. Biological organisms have safeguards or defenses against practically everything, including unnatural electromagnetic frequencies which is probably why unfamiliar EMFs trigger stress hormones.

It's not just the high frequency waves that you should concern yourself with either. Extremely low electromagnetic frequencies have been linked to increased rates of childhood leukemia, increased rates of disease, and cognitive dysfunction. Low electromagnetic frequencies were linked in 1979 by Nancy Wertheimer and Ed Leeper to the doubling of childhood leukemia rates compared to controls when in the vicinity of neighborhood distribution powerlines in Denver. The same study was repeated and confirmed in 1988 by the state of New York.

A study done in 2013 by Malka N Halgamuge (Electrical and Electronic Engineering Department, The University of Melbourne, Australia) found that wi-fi interferes with the pineal glands ability to produce melatonin. The International Agency for Research on Cancer (IARC) classifies electromagnetic fields as "possibly carcinogenic" to humans. Stating that EMFs might transform normal human cells into cancer cells. Inhibited pineal gland function has been directly connected to autism and the severity of it. Exposure to unnatural levels of EMFs is practically unavoidable for modern man due to the high utilization of electricity. How exactly these man-made EMFs influence the pineal gland is not yet known, but it is believed that the pineal gland senses EMFs as light, and as a result decreases melatonin production. This study observed the effect of exposure to weak EMFs and indicates a significant disruption in the production of melatonin which may lead to long-term negative side effects. Sleep is among the most important things we do day to day, if it is disrupted just one night, we suffer minor consequences. Imagine the effects of an entire lifetime of disrupted sleep.

Practically everywhere you go today you can hook up to free wireless wi-fi and listen to music, watch movies, download apps, call, and text someone on the other side of the planet. But at what cost? 5G is 5,000,000,000 hertz. That's the cost. 5G does not have the same range or penetration capabilities as 2.4GHz, this is the reason that so many towers are being put up so quickly. 5GHz might not be an immediate concern for humanity, because it does not penetrate walls as easily as did its lesser precursor, meaning that it may be easier to avoid if a tower isn't put on your roof. In that case, you'll want to live in a faraday cage because the cellular destruction will be quick and intense.

The frequency of 5GHZ obviously far exceeds 2.4GHz so precaution should be taken. Wi-fi has been known to disrupt the function of the pineal gland since at least 2013, this should not be taken lightly. Particularly if you enjoy sleeping, spiritual connections, altered states of consciousness, and meditation.

How many electronic conveniences do you use throughout the day? How many of them did your grandparents use? How many of these electronic conveniences did your great grandparents use? Go back to your great, great grandparents or a generation before them and I bet they didn't have one single electronic convenience. When I say convenience, I mean things as simple as switching on an electric light before the sun rises.

At this point in history, we are essentially bathing in electromagnetic radiation from wi-fi towers and cordless electrical appliances running on Bluetooth. Our phones are constantly searching for service and if it has trouble finding that service it will try harder, emitting an even higher frequency than before. Dirty electricity is another concern associated with new EMFs, dirty electricity is the basic term for electricity that can dim, change speeds, increase, or decrease function in any way. The additional pulsing from the on/off dirty electricity worsens the situation. Let's explore the history of pulsing EMFs and flickering blue lights and why we should do our best to avoid them. Especially for our children's sake.

In 1880 Thomas Edison patented the light bulb. The first and only people to enjoy artificial light for about 50 years after its invention were wealthy city people. It would take 70 years before most of the United States had access to electricity. The rural electrification project is to thank for that. As of 2016, just 13% of the world's population did not have access to electricity. Prior to 1880, 100% of the world's population didn't have electricity. The Edison bulb, or incandescent light bulb was much more like the light emitted by the sun making them much better for our biology than light bulbs today. The ability to light up the dark at that point wasn't much different than that of a fire or candle. The electricity that was needed to power the light is what changed and added high levels of constant EMFs to our life.

The television was invented in 1927 by Philo Taylor Farnsworth. It would take almost three decades until the tv found itself a permanent place in American living rooms. The first television network broadcasted from the General Electric facility in New York in January 1928. As TV progressed into a giant untapped industry businesses and media outlets found their way onto the screen and into Americans eyes and ears. In 1930 only the rich could afford televisions but by 1950 about 9% of Americans owned a TV and by 1959 85.9% of Americans owned a television. (TV History of TV Households in America: 1950-1978 Accessed November 15, 2014. http://www.tvhistory.tv/Annual_TV_Households_50-78.JPG)

This shouldn't come as a surprise as most of us probably grew up with at least one tv in our homes. According to Nielsen National Television Household on 8-8-2020 there were 121 million homes in the U.S. with TVs. They place that figure at 96.2% of homes with a connected TV set. 100 years ago, that figure was zero. That is what I call a rapid evolutionary adjustment. Humans, whom had never been subjected to blue light dominant tv images went from zero screen time to multiple hours per day and many now work in front of these screens while under compact fluorescent light bulbs that convert 60Hz AC into DC then into a higher frequency of around 50,000Hz (making fluorescent light bulbs, flickering blue-light, dirty/pulsing EMFs and in the range of damaging high frequency EMFs.)

The first complex number calculator was completed in 1940 and the world's first computer was finished by Konrad Zuse in 1941 (Computer history museum). These early computing processors though were far from personal computers as many of them took teams of people and copious amounts of space to operate. Fast forward to 1974 and Americans were buying mail-order, build-it-yourself computer kits called the Altair. They were relatively expensive, $400 at the time and not a huge hit. In 1975 the Altair BASIC was invented (by the folks that would in the same year open Microsoft) making computers much easier to use. In 1977 Apple 2 came out and made the Apple personal computer practical for all kinds of people and businesses not just hobbyists. By 1983 two million Americans owned personal computers, 54 million PCs by 1990 and that number exploded to 168 million computers by the year 2000. A survey of U.S. adults conducted January 25th through February 8th, 2021, states that about three-quarters of U.S. adults now own a desktop or laptop computer, while roughly half owned a tablet computer. Roughly 250 million or 75% of Americans had a laptop, or a desktop and 166 million, about 50% of Americans had a tablet computer. 80 years ago, those numbers were zero.

The first cell phone was invented in 1973 by Motorola. But the mobile phone didn't gain popularity until the 1990s when the price and convenience came together. In 1985 only 340,000 Americans had cellphones and by 1993 13 million, and by 1999 there were 86.1 million cell phone users, 32% of the population (The Physics Factbook). In 2005 an estimated 66% of U.S. adults had cellphones and in 2010 that number jumped to 85%. Currently that number is about 97%. The first true smart phone hit the scene in 1994 but like the cellular phone it didn't gain popularity until the price was right. The first smart phone sold as such, debuted in 2000 with a keyboard, touchscreen, and internet access. In 2007 Apples' much anticipated smart phone was unveiled and since that moment, the pockets of Americans have never be the same. Pew Research Organization puts the current number of smart phone users at 85% of the population. Not a single human owned a smart phone 30 years ago.

An article by Todd Spangler Dec. 10, 2019, states that U.S. households have an average of 11 connected devices. Seven of which having screens. In April of 2022, Parks Associates claimed that U.S. households had an average of 16 connected devices, using 63% of the previous known 7 out of 11 having screens stat, today, I expect that roughly 10 of those 16 connected devices from April 2022 had screens. In January 2019 Forbes magazine reported that the average American spends as much as 12 hours a day in front of screens. 100 years ago, human eyes had never peered into a lit screened image.

How many screens do you have in your home? Count them all. My wife and I are holistically health conscious and even we have five screens in our home. One television, two laptops and two smart phones. The television runs for about 6 hours a week give or take. We have three kiddos under six years old boogying around and we are but modern people. While I understand that in our modern world these screens and electro-magnetic frequencies cannot be entirely avoided (unless you choose to become a hermit far away from any cell tower, satellite reception and billboards) I want you to understand the side-effects of excess technology on our bodies, our planet, our energy, and our ability to connect spiritually. Awakening the

Tranquil Warrior will take diligence on every plane of your existence.

According to the Environmental Protection Agency, adults and adolescents in the United States spend 90% of their time indoors. You cannot be the best version of yourself if you spend 90% of your life indoors detached from nature and shaded from the sunshine. And no, the sunlight shining in through your window doesn't count. Windows keep out more than just wildlife. Glass blocks between 40-60% of the red-light spectrum but allows all the blue light to pass through. Red-light is good for our cells. Our atmosphere blocks much of the blue light coming from our sun, especially during sunrise and sunset when the sunlight passes through more of our atmosphere. Do you remember ROYGBIV? Red, orange, yellow, green, blue, indigo, and violet? Red light is the lowest frequency of the visible light spectrum and violet is highest i.e., Ultraviolet rays. Humanities current detachment from the outdoors, screens everywhere, unrealistic wakeful and eating hours and the lack of direct sunlight have our cells and mitochondria struggling. All the screens listed above are blue light heavy, and/or red light deprived. Much different than the natural sunlight that life on Earth evolved to utilize. Each of the 40 trillion or so cells that make up the human organism have evolved to utilize the sun and energy from the sun in some way. If humanity continues down this evolutionary path of sun and nature avoidance there's no telling what we might become but I bet, it's an ugly creature. No hair, no melanin, depleted hormones, obese, low bone density, bad eyesight, extremely low testosterone, low if any libido, lack of social skills, and little diversity (because so many people will be living in similarly simulated environments). Let's not evolve into enormous naked mole rats.

The roofs, walls, windows, and doors that keep humanity away from direct sunlight also keep us near all the screens and EMFs listed above and under artificial light for longer hours than the sun shines. This has disrupted biological function at the cellular level. Disruptions of this sort can cause dis-eases. We are energetic beings, energy is matter, energy is at the base of all emotions, all actions, all reactions, and as far as we can tell our soul itself is energy. If we intend on being capable of ferocity while remaining tranquil then we must take proper care of ourselves at the most fundamental level.

Quantum Biology is the study and application of quantum theory to aspects of biology. Quantum biology investigates the processes in biological systems that classical physics cannot answer, starting at the most basic and miniscule level that we know. Studying interactions on the quantum scale starting at quarks, electrons, protons, atoms, minerals, amino-acids, proteins, enzymes, mitochondria, and cells all the way up in scale to its effects on the entire planet, solar system, and universe. The field is uncovering powerful evidence that as biological systems advanced from the quantum level, nature, exploited the use of frequencies and vibration to create life. When you think about the previous statement it should be obvious. The laws of physics are complex and everything in existence must abide by them.

Choose sunshine over "screen time", sunlight does not flicker and is not polarized. (Sunspots on the sun do emit partially polarized light, but not directly into your eyeballs 24/7) Artificial light flickers and is polarized. Our cells are meant to receive consistent, unpolarized, non-flickering light from the sun in a cycle that goes beyond a day and night to a season-to-season cycle adapted to over thousands of years of evolution. This effects the way in which our cells receive the data from the environment. In turn, effects the way in which our cells react to the environment. When you neglect the sun, you are neglecting the needs of 40 trillion cells, these effects won't be positive.

Nature is Nurture

For all human existence we have been "grounded" at about 8.7 hertz. Today most humans reside in cities or towns with abundant electrical sources at least 50 and 60hz. This massive increase in electrical magnetic frequencies has happened in just 100 years' time. Coincidentally, excessive amounts of EMFs and the addition to copious amounts of processed sugar and seed oils began around the same time.

Roughly Three and a half billion years ago life existed at hydrothermal vents in our oceans but life on the surface was far from ready and what life did exist was barely changing or evolving. Our galaxy, the sun and atmosphere still needed to get into that "goldilocks" like state for more complex life to evolve. More than 7/8ths of our planet's history was spent in this stage known as the Precambrian period. Saying it another way, for 87.5% of Earths existence basically nothing happened in terms of evolution and biological advancement. Scientists believe that life could have just as easily stayed where it was for billions of years, but two things happened, one event about 2.1 billion years ago and the other about 570 million years ago. Researchers have claimed that 570 million years ago is when our sun began its mid-life and became stable enough for the local solar system to stabilize as well. Stars emit more ultra-violet (UV) sunlight during their mid-life than in the early or later stages. This seems to be the catalyst for life as we know it on Earth.

131

The period starting about 570 million years ago is known as the Cambrian explosion. At this point, evolution began to progress very rapidly, single celled organisms evolving and co-evolving into multi-celled organisms across the planet. Many new species evolved quickly, gaining size and complexity leading to a wide variety of life. For the Cambrian explosion to begin something else had to happen at the cellular level.

One cell engulfed another cell, both cells survived symbiotically, one of which using the other as a power source, or maybe the other way around. One cell (mitochondria) learned to use the other for protection and mobilization? Either way this harmonized coevolution led to animal life as we know it today. Mitochondria and sun light are a key piece to this evolutionary puzzle and thus, obviously a key piece to overall human health.

Roughly 2.1 billion years ago this special and rare circumstance occurred. Nothing happened for 1.5 billion years after that coevolution. Prokaryotic cells evolve quickly but never into complex organisms like eukaryotic cells do. It could have been a fluke, coincidence, Aliens, fate, God, I don't know, but I am grateful for this event, and you should be too.

Eukaryotic cells appeared after two prokaryotic cells became one functioning organism. One of which becoming what we now know as the mitochondria. This is important because all complex life that we see on earth contains these eukaryotic cells. You, me, that spider in the corner, the trees, the mushrooms growing in the shade along with the moss and algae all share incredibly similar traits at the microscopic level. Prior to this cooperative evolution the mitochondria were their own species, receiving information in the form of frequencies, perceiving that information, and then adapting to that environment. Mitochondria continue to do this today, EMFs have them on high alert more often than they can handle, contributing to cardiovascular disease on a large scale. Mitochondrial health is one of the most basic yet important components of overall health.

The brain and the heart contain the most mitochondria in the body, they are the power source of the cells. The gut is also loaded with these power houses. Have you ever heard someone say we have two brains? Or maybe three brains? Due to the high number of mitochondria in the brain, heart and gut it's easy to make the connection. What all places can we "think" from? We have "gut reactions", make decisions from our heart, and of course use our brain. When our mitochondrial health is supreme all three of these "brains" work in coherence and we become limitless, tranquil warriors as evolution intended.

The result of mitochondrial function is ATP (adenosine triphosphate). Mitochondria are light converters inside our cells. Some cells like red blood cells have no mitochondria and other cells like the ones in our brain or heart can have more than 5,000 mitochondria per cell. Mitochondria are basically alchemists, using a very special function called the electron chain transfer. This process is the movement of electrons that go through a chain of events, the electrons, based on their complexity, are converted into elements and then chemicals. Essentially this is a conversion of light into matter, various types of matter. Mitochondria takes these light molecules and creates elements and chemicals. They also create water, which acts as a battery and a conductive medium for the electrical chain of events. Our brains and our hearts are the most electromagnetic parts of the human body due to this process. Brains and hearts function essentially from light. Therefore, we can shock the heart or the mitochondria in the heart to restart it after a malfunction or heart attack. "Clear! Bzzz!"

Bruce Lipton, Author and PHD estimates that the human body has at least 3.5 trillion volts, that's trillion with a T. The average lightning strike contains just 15 million volts. Your body contains about 233,333 lightning strikes at any given moment. Basically, you're Thor. You are a walking bolt of lightning, two hundred and thirty-three thousand of them. Cellular health matters, can you see how important it is now?

What does all this mean concerning blue lights, EMFs, and the technology that produce them? Blue light, electromagnetic frequencies that differ from our natural state provided by mother earth and the sun affect the way our cell's function, in a harmful way. Your smart phone is between four hundred fifty million and two billion seven hundred million hertz, quite a bit different that mother earths 8.7Hz. The distance that the EMF radiation can travel varies widely but you can rest assure that while your smart phone is on your body it is sending heavy amounts of cell damaging waves into you. There are many different types of EMFs around us daily which is why it is important to limit exposure while we are at our homes. Cell towers have been shown to be the most destructive as the frequencies they produce are incredibly high and penetrate through homes easily and the new style (5G) is very high, although less penetrative. If you know that you live near a cell tower, I suggest purchasing a few in home EMF blocking devices and spend as much time "grounded" in direct contact with the Earth or on a grounding matt as possible. If you can find a source of natural water to swim or soak in, do it often! Clean and natural bodies of water are loaded with minerals, elements, and charged ions that make it a great conductor of electricity.

Meaning that when you are swimming in a clean lake, river, ocean etc., all the parts of you touching the water are grounding, not just the bottoms of your feet when your barefoot. The benefits of barefoot grounding are impeccable, now imagine it from head to toe, hydrostatic pressure pushing the grounding qualities into places you could never put into direct contact with the earth.

Mitochondria uses the energy absorbed by the cell and electrons from light and *food* that absorbed that light to carry out its conversions. When we take away the natural sun light and replace it with this bastardized, flickering blue light, we are throwing off the way in which the mitochondria are designed to function. When you create dis-ease in trillions of powerhouses in your body you will surely notice dis-ease on a large scale. Check out the work of Jack Kruse for an even deeper rabbit hole into these issues.

What can improve or restore human mitochondrial function to that of our early ancestors? Begin exposing your skin to natural sun light with-out the use of sunscreen, sunglasses, and excess clothing. Eating plants grown organically in the amount of sunlight they require. Eating animals raised in conditions equal to that of their natural habitat, in the amount of sun they would naturally receive, and eating an ancestrally consistent diet. Eating mushrooms under those same conditions, grown where they have evolved to grow, consuming the nutrients they were designed to, and being exposed to the amount of sunlight they require.

One of my favorite ways to improve health at the mitochondrial level is the most difficult for some people. Get chilly. Brrrr! Cold increase's mitochondrial function and speed because it condenses the electron chain transfer process, the electron or light can make more trips in less time. The cold does some truly amazing things for your entire body, and we will explore more of the submerged part of that iceberg later. Maybe you're afraid of plunging into cold water, I get it, perhaps you'd give it a chance if you could enjoy a hot cacao afterwards? Cacao contains pyrroloquinoline quinone (PQQ) and this chemical causes mitochondrial genesis. This means It increases the number of mitochondria in the body by activating genes that oversee mitochondrial protection, reproduction, and repair. You can also eat foods containing DHA. Like egg yolks, liver, walnuts, and wild-caught salmon. DHA is known to contribute to the effectiveness of the mitochondria.

Artificial light distorts mitochondrial function. Each human cell (besides red blood cells) can have anywhere from 2 to 5,000 mitochondria. The human organism is made up of about 40 trillion cells. Some estimates suggest that each neuron in the brain can have up to 2 million mitochondria and the human brain has about 86 billion neurons. The heart itself has about 40,000 neurons and a total of 2 to 3 billion cells. The number of mitochondria in our brains and hearts are staggering, and hard to estimate due to genetic, lifestyle and health differences between people. Regardless of genetics, or current health status you need to improve your mitochondrial and cellular function today, unless you don't care to live a longer, more productive, tranquil, able, and joyful life. If our heart has the second most mitochondria in our bodies, then we need to look at mitochondrial health more closely when considering cardiovascular diseases. Cardiac diseases are the two leading causes of death and the number of lives they take yearly is increasing.

My practically free prescription: get your naked skin in the sunshine daily, take an ice bath or cold shower at least three times a week, drink a hot fresh cacao without processed sugar, and eat some salmon, eggs, and liver at least two times a week. Increasing mitochondrial health will positively increase your overall health. Quickly. Sunshine is FREE so utilize the heck out of that script whenever possible.

Leptin is a hormone that suppresses hunger, accelerates metabolic rate, and provides long-term energy. Leptin is produced in adipose (fat) tissue where it is sent into the circulatory system, making its way to the hypothalamus gland in the brain. The brain gets the signal and then sends a signal to the body that you've had enough to eat. Research shows that obese people are leptin resistant because of overeating, specifically the over-consumption of processed sugar. Which results in the hypothalamus becoming less sensitive to leptin. Separate studies have also shown that sleep deprivation can cause a resistance to leptin. This one I know to be true, I spent many years working on three to four hours of sleep and can attest to the cravings associated with increased leptin resistance.

Leptin's complementing hormone, ghrelin, is secreted by the stomach and increases hunger. Like leptin, ghrelin enters the bloodstream on its way to the hypothalamus. Sleep deprivation increases ghrelin levels and decreases leptin. High levels of insulin in the blood can inhibit leptin and increase ghrelin as well.

Tying this back to light. There are a few things that adequate sunlight does when concerning these hormones. Making you more sensitive to leptin and consequently less sensitive to ghrelin. This is a good thing; you want to be more sensitive to leptin and less sensitive to ghrelin so that you feel less hunger. Subsequently eating less. Sunlight increases levels of Vitamin D, which decreases the level of proinflammatory cytokines, cytokines are the hormones that cause inflammation. Decreasing those makes you more sensitive to Leptin.

To control hunger at the quantum level first, get naked(ish) in the sun every day. Secondly, get rid of or limit as much emf and blue light exposure as possible. Thirdly, get a good night's rest. Fourthly, stop eating copious amounts of un-natural sugars, or flat out stop. Finally, enjoy a better life untethered to the fridge.

Blocking Blue Light and Changing Your Tech Habits

Natural blue-light from the suns light spectrum is beneficial during the day because it boosts mood, attention, and reaction times. But during the night these benefits aren't so beneficial. Blue light affects sleep and may cause several diseases. Until the invention of the light bulb the sun was the major source of light and there was no such thing as a light that shined in the blue spectrum after hours. Now in most of the world the darkest part of the day is spent under a spectrum of light that would have only been observed during the brightest times of the mid-day. This may contribute to cancer, diabetes, heart disease, and obesity.

The modern workspace requires that many people work indoors under flickering blue lights, void of natural sun light and possibly in front of screens for the better part of their shift. My recent career was outdoors and in front of a screen. All my reporting and calculations were done on a screen, my communicating and recording were done in this manner as well. Although I spent about half of my 12 hour long shift out in the environment, the other half of my shift was spent staring into a screen. I was lucky enough to be able to escape the screen for long periods throughout the day. Many workers today don't have that option and yet 50 years ago, this problem did not exist.

Working in front of flickering blue lights for long periods of time have been linked to depression, anxiety, diminished vision (peripheral too), and social communication issues.

Young children become easily addicted to screens and it's no wonder when you consider how hyperactive their imaginations are. The screen provides ideas, constructs, and characters to fuel more imaginations. But, so does the forest, the lake, ocean etc. The side effects that are observed in adults from excessive screen time, emfs, and lack of sun exposure are miniscule when compared to the destruction done to little developing brains, eyes, organs, and personalities.

Here are a few ways to avoid and limit exposure to EMFs and blue light without moving to a currently uninhabited island. Put your Wi-fi box behind a concrete wall, or behind walls period. Don't run the Wi-fi 24/7 if you don't need to, turn your phones off or on airplane mode whenever possible (especially while sleeping), and purchase emf blockers for each room where people will be sleeping. Get rid of your multi-speed fan, change your dimming light fixtures, and limit the use of any appliance that has differing outputs or speeds. Get rid of your microwave. Purchase blue-light blocking glasses and screen protectors for your cellphones, tablets, and computer screens. They are relatively cheap and come in practically every size. Beware that it will change the way colors look on these devices. Screen adhesives for televisions are harder to find but they are becoming more popular as more people learn about the topic.

While typing this book, I have a blue-light blocker on my computer screen and went into the settings and removed as much of the blue light spectrum as I could. I also set it on night mode from 8pm to 8am to eliminate the extra blue lights while still being able to see my screen while the sun was shining.

Set limits for yourself and your children. No screens before or after a certain time, be consistent and diligent about your times. For almost three years our children believed that our television didn't work when the sun was shining, or at night-time. Hey, we lie about Santa, the Easter bunny, tooth fairy, why not lie about something that will elevate them? Instead of turning on the TV, show them how to build forts, climb trees, throw rocks, dig holes, whatever just get them using their imagination instead of borrowing it from the boob tube and its compadres.

A real hippy-dippy thing you can do is to unplug entirely. Yeah, whoa, crazy idea, right? Live like a human being? No googling shit you don't need to know. No arguing with someone on Facebook because you disagree with their post. No binge-watching Netflix. No mindless scrolling. I know, I know. Crazy! Instead of all those mindless habits you can replace them (even if just for a few hours a day) with reading, walking, laying in the grass, sunbathing, lifting heavy shit, stretching, breathwork, hiking, journaling, gardening, petting an animal, or meditating. Read or listen to "The Three-Day Effect" by Florence Williams, "Forest Bathing" by Dr. Qing Li, "EMF'd" by Dr. Joseph Mercola, or "Earthing" by Martin Zucker for some motivation on why you may want to consider some time unplugged. Another sensual idea is lighting candles in the evening and shutting off the electrical lights. Flame lit light and incandescent are the most similar to sunlight. Use candles with minimal or no artificial fragrances and harmful chemicals since you will be breathing it in.

How to Tan and Use Sunshine to be Better at Everything

Being tan is a sign of vitality. If you are eating an adequate diet that promotes healthy cellular function and listen to signs from your skin like sun burn, blisters etc. the sun is going to benefit you, not harm you. Skin cancer is triggered internally. When a doctor tells you to avoid sunshine and lather harmful chemicals on your skin if you must be in the sun, you should tell them to stick their stethoscope where the sun doesn't shine and then, go find yourself a new doctor. Mitochondria require near infra-red light from the sun for optimal function. Taking a daily vitamin and hoping to reach your daily requirements for Vitamin D is like trying to store water in a strainer. Vitamin D is a hormone and your body needs sunlight, specifically from the red-light spectrum to synthesize it. Ever since our first ancestor walked out into the grasslands about 2 million years ago, we started living in direct sunlight and evolved to utilize it. We shed most of our body hair and replaced it with sweat glands. Simultaneously increased melanin in our skin, kept hair on the tops of our heads like natural hats, hair around our reproductive organs to assist in sun protection and learned to utilize our environment when the sun was too much to tolerate. As humanity trekked into new hemispheres where the spectrum of light and climates were different, skin tone adapted. Clothes were more necessary in colder climates, further lessening the need for melanin and adjusting pigmentation to better suit the environment.

Melanin provides the pigmentation of your skin, eyes, and hair. It also absorbs harmful UV rays to protect other cells from UV ray damage. Melanin is produced by melanocytes and all humans are assumed to have roughly the same number of melanocytes, but the amount of melanin each one produces, and the pigmentation of the melanin depend on your consistent exposure to sunlight and your genetics. Eumelanin provides black and brown skin, eyes, and hair. The closer to the equator your recent ancestors evolved, the more eumelanin will be produced vs pheomelanin. Pheomelanin provides a more reddish tone, it is responsible for the pigmentation of our lips, nipples, and private regions with reddish tones. People with more pheomelanin tend to tan more red than brown or black and people with equal amounts of pheomelanin and eumelanin have red hair. Clusters of melanocytes result in freckles, most common in people with Northern European ancestry. The more time you spend in the sun, the more melanin your body will produce. Melanin keeps ultra-violet rays from damaging your DNA by redistributing the rays to the outer layers of the skin.

The more melanin you have, the less sunlight gets deep into your skin. This was problematic for ancestral populations that moved farther from the equator and for clothed populations. Thus, populations further from the equator saw changes in skin tone. This was problematic because although the brisk cold warranted the protection of some outer wear, we still needed to absorb sunlight for energy. Hence the lighter complexion. Researchers and archeologists agree that populations around the world even in the northern European region were plenty darker than their present-day relatives. Take Eskimos as an example of a more homeostatic complexion for ancestral hunter-gatherers. The addition of clothes, subtraction of bioavailable and highly nutritious animal foods, addition of large quantities of plant foods, and of course more time spent indoors led to the more dramatic changes we see in skin tone today. Researchers suggest that this dramatic shift in skin tone might be less than 4,000 years old, about the time that agriculture took the drivers seat around the world. People around the planet cover their bodies with clothing and the tiny parts that are exposed to sun they lather in harsh chemicals in fear that the sun is going to hurt them. This is leading to an even lighter complexion overall as our bodies desperately try to evolve.

People with more melanin need more sun exposure to achieve optimal health, on the other hand people with less melanin need less exposure to achieve optimal health. Meaning that people with a lot of melanin are susceptible to deficiencies and the health concerns that come with when they migrate to hemispheres with less intense sun exposure, think African descendants in Canada and the high inclination towards obesity, diabetes, and CVD. Conversely people from those climates with less intense sun exposure experience the harmful side effects of UV radiation when they move to hemispheres with more intense sun exposure, think European descendants in Australia and the high inclination for skin cancer, melanoma, and basal-cell carcinoma. Both groups are susceptible to diseases and DNA damage. Excess sun exposure poses risks, but the risks are much more tolerable than what lack of exposure will inflict.

The fragile skulls found at Pelusium. Herodotus a Greek historian recalls his witness to the skulls of defeated soldiers from the battle of Pelusium, in which the Persian King Cambyses defeated the Egyptians in 525 BCE. Herodotus notices that the skulls of Persian soldiers are so weak that hitting them with a small pebble will make a hole in them. While the

Egyptian skulls were so thick that with a large stone they would hardly break. The cause of it he believed was "namely that the Egyptians beginning from their early childhood shave their heads, and the bone is thickened by exposure to the sun; and this is also the cause of their not becoming bald-headed; for among Egyptians, you see fewer bald-headed men than among any other race. This then is the reason why these have their skulls strong; and the reason why the Persians have theirs weak is that they keep them delicately in the shade from the first by wearing tiaras, that is felt caps."

Today, people of all races are becoming balder, fatter, paler, and less happy because (amongst a multitude of factors) they are avoiding the sun's rays. Vitamin D levels are at all time low, testosterone is dropping dramatically every generation, bone density is decreasing, skeletal muscle is wasting away, and yet people are bombarded with ads and misinformation regarding the easiest and cheapest way to improve all those issues. Sunshine! Its FREE and its available every single day! Even through the clouds.

Still don't believe that sunshine is good for you, fine, here are some more reasons to utilize the sun to optimize health. Sunlight boosts serotonin. Serotonin gives you more sustainable energy, keeps you tranquil, focused, and more positive. Sunlight increases testosterone levels, which in turn increases fertility and libido in both men and women. Testosterone also makes your waist slimmer, muscles bigger, bones denser, and immune function more optimal. UV rays also have anti-bacterial, anti-viral, and germicidal qualities, our natural microbiome is proficient in handling sun exposure but many of the germs and viruses that infect us today are not equipped to handle UV radiation, a sunbath is better for your than a bubble bath.

Sunlight helps improve sleep by setting your circadian rhythm and triggering the production of melatonin, better sleep equates to better everything. Sunlight stimulates the production of vitamin D, which is an essential hormone that supports bone health, lower blood pressure, increased metabolic function, supports efficient mineral absorption, reduces depression, supports immune function, reduces the risk of autoimmune diseases, and maintains muscle mass while reducing adipose fat storage. Sun exposure has also been observed to extend your life.

How to begin utilizing the sun's rays to massively improve your wellbeing if you have sensitive skin. Begin with the sunrise and sunset rays, spending some leisure time with a lot of skin exposed before 10am and after 6pm. During these hours the sunlight must travel through more obstructions to get to your skin, the atmosphere blocks and protects us from much of the damaging solar rays. Try *sun-gazing,* a practice where you literally gaze at the sun, with your eyes closed. I incorporate this with my morning meditation practice, just face the horizon with your eyes shut, gazing at the sun beyond your eyelids. This will reset your circadian rhythm and signal to your cells to begin producing daytime hormones and prepares your skin to absorb beneficial UV rays and defend against the harmful ones. If you have pale or sensitive skin, you want to avoid the mid-day sun because the UV rays are traveling through less atmosphere to get to you and much more of the blue-light spectrum that is damaging gets through. Don't stop living your life when the sun is high, just put on a hat, or some clothing, let your skin build a tolerance and mindfully notice when you need to add clothes, find shade, or hydrate. Try increments of no more than 5-15 minutes with most of your naked body exposed until you feel comfortable in your skins ability to handle the mid-day sun and then increase your exposure time. Hydration is a big part of avoiding skin damage in excessive sunlight. If you are eating ancestrally then you are already a step ahead and will experience much less sun damage because you are consuming adequate minerals and nutrients. Add some fruits and extra cups of mineralized water on days that you know you'll be in the sun more often. *Especially* days that you will be drinking and in the sun all day, alcohol seems to impair your skin's ability to gauge the power of the suns rays, making you more vulnerable. Additional minerals and nutrients will help with that. (Mineralized water is water with added minerals, specifically minerals like zinc, manganese, magnesium, iron, iodine, potassium, calcium, copper, selenium, and phosphorus.)

As a minor precaution, we made a mistake a few years ago with our children that we will never make again. A spring vacation to somewhere a dozen hours south, reflective sand and water, with very little full body sunshine preparation, no preparedness with umbrellas, no sunscreen, no long sleeves, and a few hours in the high noon sun is a bad story. They kids got very bad sun burns and we learned a valuable lesson that I am passing on to you now. We do this now as a family, during the winter months we all go outside every day and expose at least 25% of our skin to direct sunlight. Sometimes it takes intervals because it's so cold, but we do it anyways, this became a practice partly for sun exposure and partly for cold exposure. If we are planning an early spring vacation, we pack long sleeve sun shirts and hats for us and the kids, bring some shade and make sure that we are ultra-hydrating and eating extra bone marrow all week prior.

A new popular trend has immerged where people are touting the benefits of tanning their perineum's (the space between your anus and your gender identifier). Mainstream science seems to be very harshly against this practice, for me, that warrants it as a worthy thing to attempt. I have not, although being naked in the sun is 100% the most energizing thing you can do so the tanning of your nether regions has verifiable results. Your perineum is your root chakra, your most primal energy center and the health of this energy center is extremely important, physically, mentally, and spiritually. But the butt in the sun trend is untested as far as I am aware. The skin there is sensitive compared to elsewhere on the body and ancestrally it does make sense that your *taint* would get direct sunshine from time to time, but not prolonged exposure. If you have the place and time to try it just use caution.

Social Dilema, I Mean Media, Social Media

Social media consumes a ton of precious time. Time that you cannot get back. Americans spend an average of 147 minutes per day on social media sites (from Statista.com). While it is nice to check in on distant friends and family and to keep up to date with the ongoings of people you care about it can become a detrimental issue in your life. Constantly "checking in on" hundreds, or thousands of people that you may or may not actually know. Then of course you must let all your "followers" know what you are up to. You compete with their posts for popularity, compare yourself to their pictured "life". You like their posts, they like yours or maybe they don't, the anxiety of how many likes you did or didn't get, how many views, how many reactions, the anxiety of comparing yourself to everyone else gets a whole lot more complicated when you have the entire world to compare yourself against. I didn't have to go through puberty or adolescence with social media and I am thankful for that, just imagine how incredibly insane that must be for a teenager today. Thousands of images of fully "developed" women and men to compare themselves against. People from around the world. I only had to concern myself with the people in my town.

As a personal trainer and self-proclaimed health nut I had always felt the need to build a community using social media platforms. This "need" created unnecessary stress in my life. The stress of grammar, spelling, 100% factual, non-offensive, and inarguable information, photo quality, political correctness, the timing, and then of course the anxiety about how people will or won't react. What the internet has named "trolls" are everywhere and if I post a picture of something or say something that some troll doesn't agree with, they attack. It happens to a lot of people, all the time and it's stressful. Bottom line is this, social media addiction is real, its psychologically destructive and you should do your best to control your time on it. I often detach entirely from social media for weeks at a time. I only use Facebook and Instagram; I get on Facebook maybe once a month, but Instagram I generally get on once a day for about 30-45 minutes during the times that I am not social media "fasting". Young teens are more susceptible to the addiction and negative side-effects of over consuming social media, if you can keep your kids from these platforms I recommend doing so before they manipulate their innocence, perception of their body, perception of love and friendship.

Excessive screen time is connected to lack of outdoor time, and excessive sedentary time which in turn is connected to excessive adipose tissue. In other words, screens contribute to obesity. Turning off your screens will allow you to explore your own dreams and goals while using your own innate intelligence. You will be surprised what you are truly capable of when you stop gawking over what everyone else is capable of. Get off the couch and move, specifically outdoors in the sunshine.

Breaking the addiction to screens can be as easy as adding meaningful face-to-face interactions into your daily life or it can be like breaking a drug addiction. When you receive a positive notification from someone on your smartphone you get a little hit of dopamine, the more notifications you receive, the more dopamine hits you get. Face to face interactions can help a lot when trying to overcome this addiction. Join a group or class of like-minded people and make some friends.

CHAPTER FIVE

CLEAN FREAKS AND MICROBIOME TERRORISM

Insane sanitation, this is something that many of us may have had a chance to evaluate during the recent immune system crisis. Squirts of microbiome killing sanitizer everywhere, bleach and biocide splashed on everything in hopes of eliminating something that ultimately could not be eradicated through such methods. All the meanwhile inflicting horrible havoc on our endocrine and immune systems worsening the situation.

Ultra-sanitation inevitably leads to weakened immune systems. We all know this, just like Grandpa and Grandma used to say about the children, "let em play in the dirt, it's good for em!" Because it's true. Or when you got hurt as a kid "Rub some dirt on it!" Right? Maybe I was just lucky to hear those words when I was bleeding profusely and crying about an open wound. Truthfully, an immune system that is in coherence with its environment is an optimal immune system. I wouldn't go rubbing dirt on a wound deeper than your average sidewalk scrape, user discretion is advised.

Exposing ourselves to germs and the natural environment increases our body's ability to defend itself. The cells involved in our defenses remember enemies and save that information from battle to battle so that if they encounter that foe or a similar foe, they know how to eliminate, use, or moderate it.

Kids kept in bubbles deal with more allergies, illnesses, and diseases than kids raised smushing their toes around in the mud surrounded by other people and animals in nature.

Our immune system is arguably the most complex system in the body because it includes every part of us. From our skin microbiome, our mouth microbiome, our genital microbiome, the microbes on our eye lashes, eyebrows, to the microbes living deep in our intestines, each population of microbes living in a biome that is perfect for them. Even our perception of the environment in which we reside plays a role. Energetically speaking our aura plays a large role in keeping us healthy as well, working as an energetic immune system. When it is weak, we are weak, and when it's strong, we are as well.

Some of our micro-immune warriors aren't *ours* at all, they are hired guns and mercenaries. What I mean is that they aren't our human cells, although they live in harmony inside and/or on us serving us this defensive purpose while we feed them and give them a comfortable home, they are hitchhikers. Some of which we got from Momma at birth, (skin to skin, Vaginal birth, breast feeding etc.) and some of which we picked up from our environment, diet, and lifestyle. Co-evolution of micro-organisms hitching rides helped to strengthen our immune system and gave these organisms a thriving environment. We give them a cozy environment to live, and they will defend that environment with their lives. When we douse ourselves in bacteria killing substances, we are destroying our own little defensive army and damaging their habitat at the same time.

If you're not taking suitable care of those micro-organisms' habitat (your body) their performance will decline. Foes start to look like friends and friends start to look like foes, they are destined to defend and destroy but will have a difficult time figuring out who the real enemy is. This goes for human immune cells and the hired guns. Eventually they can attack the human body. Leading to inflammation and auto-immune diseases like arthritis.

If our microbiome gets knocked out of symbiosis it will be in dis-symbiosis meaning they will not be living in harmony. There are a multitude of ways in which we damage our micro-biomes across our entire body, as we mentioned previously eating processed sugar disrupts and damages our bodies a ton, and one of the most harmful ways it does is by disrupting our gut micro-biome, leading to hormonal imbalances, inadequate or excessive release of certain hormones that lead to even harsher imbalances and inadequacies that eventually destroy the entire human organism. This destruction of the microbiome leaves many people open to harmful infections. The cycle worsens as the body gets weaker and weaker. When we take anti-biotics (against life) or use antibacterial products (against bacteria) we wreck our microbiome. What you consume both through your mouth and skin contribute to or take away from your overall health. TAKE CARE OF YOUR TOMB. And in turn, it will take care of you.

Train your immune system by utilizing your terrain. This starts at birth, babies born vaginally, breast fed, given lots of "skin to skin" contact (Mom, Dad, and siblings), raised with siblings, raised outdoors in the sun and grass, around animals, and allowed to explore their environment will have a stronger immune system than a baby born C-section, bottle fed from birth, raised alone, and in a sanitized bubble. That's just the truth. Maximizing microbial contact in children is better than any inoculation.

Young children, toddlers, and infants have impeccable immune memory. Meaning that the microbes they encounter will be permanently engrained in their immune defense headquarters. Some evidence suggests that these antibodies can even be passed down to their children. As we age our immune system tends to hang onto antibodies for shorter durations. This varies widely from person to person depending on their overall health and how much time they spend exposing themselves to… well life.

If your parents let you play outside and brought you to your cousins' house when they found out they had chicken pox just so you could get it too, let you play in the mud, sand, dirt, soil, or other "unsanitary" places, or if your parents let you eat some food off the ground abiding by the "three second rule" or watched you eat a booger or let the dog lick your face when you were little, believe it or not, they were actually helping you. This may sound like an early stage of neglect, but truth is, kids raised in the environment, can defend themselves against their environment. If you were neglected enough to develop a robust immune system, take a moment to thank your parents now.

Don't worry if you weren't raised that way though because the immune system is ever evolving and adjusting. Don't worry if you haven't been raising your children that way either, again, the immune system is always evolving and adjusting. You can always start now with these behaviors. Go outside barefoot every single day. Spend time every day in direct sunshine minus the sunscreen, sunglasses, and excess clothing. Breathe in the fresh air daily. Winter, spring, summer or fall all you've got to do is call, nature. Pet an animal, pet lots of animals. Eat foods that are anti-inflammatory. Sleep at a consistent time every night and wake up at a consistent time with a smile every morning.

Twist and move daily to let your lymph system function properly. Doing this will allow it to remove toxins more effectively from your body. Exercise 3-5 times a week minimally, in moderate to intense bouts consisting of 30-60 minutes. Stay active outside of those bouts as well, setting a step goal can help keep you accountable. Don't over-eat, fast sometimes, eat only when the sun is out and be happy. Do what we talked about in the previous chapter with negating the effects of blue light and your immune system will skyrocket to Marvels' Wolverine status. Avoid fear, choose faith. Avoid frowning, choose smiling. Avoid guilt, choose pride. Avoid jealousy and choose hope.

About Petting Pets

Having a pet around can improve immunity at the microbial level, can reduce stress at a psychological level, and dogs can even detect dis-ease in humans. Did you know there are dogs specifically trained to smell high blood sugar in diabetics? Dogs can also smell cancer and other diseases early on in humans even if they have never been around this person before to develop a memory of that individual's scent.

One time while my parents were over visiting, Stetson, our blue heeler wouldn't leave my mom alone. He kept sniffing and poking around near her one armpit and chest. He got shooed away, by me and my mom, as most people do when a dog won't leave a guest alone. He didn't seem upset or like he was really trying to signal anything to us, but he was very curious about a scent he was picking up. She was diagnosed with breast cancer just a few weeks after that incident. We like to joke that Stetson; our blue heeler is a blue *healer.*

Dogs can pick up the scent of what are called volatile organic compounds or VOCs for short. VOCs are carbon containing chemicals that are more complex than CO2. They are excreted from our breath, phlegm, urine, and skin. These chemical signals and scents reflect our internal health, particular diseases have specific chemical scents that dogs pick up. Dogs have an amazing olfactory system, but many nurses swear that they can smell a patient that has a late-stage cancer or Parkinson's disease.

This is where we can get into the part about body-odor. If I'm suggesting that people need to do less sanitizing and cleaning, I need to address the smelly individuals in the room. Why do people get so stinky in the first place? If dogs can smell disease in a human and can signal to human beings that something is wrong due to that smell, (I believe cats and other domesticated animals that live around humans can also do the same thing it just hasn't been observed as far as I know). I also believe that humans although maybe at a lesser capacity have the same ability.

I have been eating an ancestrally consistent diet as well as I can in the modern world for about three years now. I shower about five times a week in the winter, and maybe two to three times a week in the summer. As odd as it sounds, in the summer months I "stink" less. During the summer I expose more of my skin to direct sunlight for longer periods of time and practically all the plant foods I eat come from our garden or from a local farm. Whereas in the winter months where more of the plant foods come from further away, I expose myself to direct sunlight less, and spend less time overall barefoot. While I still practice what I preach and expose my skin to direct sunlight for at least 30 minutes per day with no shirt on, and ground barefoot no matter the weather, that is nothing compared to the hours on end that I spend this way during the summer months. I believe this has a lot to do with the increase in body-odor during winter. During the summer months I obviously sweat more often so you would assume that I would stink more, but I don't. Common knowledge is that human health declines in the winter months and I believe lack of sunlight is the biggest reason for this. Therefore, the winter stink is more prevalent, but it's not what it used to be. There was a time in my late teenage years and early 20's where I remember lathering my pits with harmful deodorant several times a day. All while showering once in the morning, once after gym class, and a third time after sports practice or games. Yet the B.O. was still there. Now, I can work out, do a sauna session, work, and still not stink by the end of the day. For a few days at least in the summer. In the winter, like I said it comes sooner. I only use deodorant on special occasions now like holiday family gatherings, long trips and "date days" with my lovely wife.

When you increase or restore your health, you decrease the negative body odor. Speaking from an evolutionary standpoint, humans in hunting and gathering communities of 150 or so members would pick up on one anothers smells or VOCs quickly. Especially since cleanliness was practically non-existent. Considering that most of the animals our ancestors hunted have fantastic olfactory senses they would have easily picked up on the scent of a stinky human, making it difficult to provide a successful hunt. I believe body odor is one of the true first signals of disease in the human body. Think of times in your life when you were the unhealthiest or times after you ate a very unhealthy meal, your *secretions* weren't pleasant were they? Even to the untrained and un-impressive human nose these scents are detectable. Just like nurses who claim they can "smell" cancer and Parkinson's disease, imagine what you could detect in the body odors around you if you tried.

Humans function outside of our biological intelligence often and this great and wonderful consciousness we possess makes us second guess our innate responses repeatedly. We often realize that "something" just isn't right, but we rarely give it much more attention than that.

Bumblebees have stinky feet just like people. Okay maybe not "just" like people. But their feet leave behind a trail of chemical scents signaling to other bumblebees where they have been. Leading them to food sources or back to the hive. There is no question that some people's feet can stink to high Heaven and could definitely leave behind a trail. But the purpose doesn't seem to be the same. Humans were barefoot for practically all our existence minus the last few thousand years. Up until the past century though these shoes were made from natural sources, i.e., plants, and animals. Today they are made from synthetic materials that are particularly unhealthy for us (and separate our electrical energy from the earth). A barefoot ancestor would have encountered many scratches and scrapes on their feet, leaving them vulnerable to deadly infection. Yet evidence shows this to be an extremely rare scenario. Without shoes then what was protecting their feet? Micro-soldiers in the form of a microbiome. The natural foot micro-biome hosts a species of micro-organisms that are lethal to certain types of fungus and other species. They are essentially elite defensive warriors, like the navy seals, or army rangers of the immune system.

Today though, humans clean their feet with harsh chemicals (killing these micro-warriors and their habitat), cover their feet in synthetic socks, then a synthetic shoe, they rarely place their bare feet directly on the earth's surface, they don't let their feet ever see sun light, thus, leaving their feet vulnerable to athletes' foot amongst other funguses and infections and making them "stinkier" than ever before.

Do yourself and your feet a favor, get them in the sunshine and in direct contact with the ground. Your immune system will appreciate it, and you might even lessen the stench from your gym sneakers.

The Nature of Cleanliness

Cleanliness is necessary for all animals but to what extent? Just yesterday morning I was sitting in the woods, it was about 7:30am, first light was just creeping in, I was sitting on a log waiting on a monster buck to bless me with a broad side shot to fill our freezer when I started hearing some splashing and swimming in the stream about 5yds from the log I was sitting on. I could barely make out what it was until the sun came up a bit more. Two musk rats splashing around like a couple of kids. They were having a blast chasing each other around, it almost looked like they were playing tag in the water. I watched and admired them for a bit as the rest of the animals in the forest began to liven up. After a bit I had seen several squirrels, chipmunks, a blue herring, ducks, blue jays, cardinals, a hawk, few crows, chickadees, chipmunks, rabbits, a doe, and of course the musk rats, but no monster buck. I noticed something about them all as I silently observed. They ALL cleaned themselves. The muskrats got up on shore shortly after their game and cleaned themselves off with their paws, then came to one another's assistance to clean those hard-to-reach places. I watched each one of these animals clean themselves off in one way or another that day. I often watch our ducks at the house clean themselves both in the water and out, and of course our dog, but it never really occurred to me how often and for what reasons until I began writing this chapter.

I wonder how much of this twisting, scraping, scrubbing, rinsing, and picking is necessary for proper lymph flow, which I would argue is an important part of cleanliness. Internally. And I wonder how much of all that has to do with external cleanliness. And why did all these animals clean so thoroughly? They don't need to look pretty for one another, do they?

To a large extent the outward appearance of an animal gives its potential mate an intimate look at their health and genetic capacity for survival. The ability to remain clean of debris, dirt, grime, bugs etc. shows proper health. It also lets a would-be predator know their health status. Being uncleanly can make an animal look like a weak and easy target. Many woodland creatures must deal with constant bombardment and harassment by ticks, fleas and the like. Constant and consistent picking, scraping, scrubbing, and rinsing aid in that battle. Cleanliness appears to be necessary for survival to a certain extent.

Is there such thing as over sanitation? Where should we draw the line? We know that our ancestral relatives (the period spanning from 2 million to 20k years ago) suffered very little, if ever from diseases. They never smeared trolamine salicylate, PABA, avobenzone, oxybenzone, octocrylene, homosalate, octisalate, or octinoxate on their skin to *protect* them from the sun. They never washed their largest organ with microplastics, parabens, sodium laureth sulfate, sodium laurel sulfate, triclosan, triclocarban, phthalates, mineral oil, retinyl, formaldehyde, or toluene. They didn't brush their teeth with fluoride and propylene glycol (the main ingredient in anti-freeze.) So, yeah, I think there is such a thing as over sanitation. Each of the chemicals listed above has its own dangers, but in the chemical concoctions we call soaps, or cleansers the dangers are multiplied. Many of them disrupt hormones and damage the central nervous system.

Ancestrally, humans did bathe, they did use sun-blocks when needed and they did sanitize. They bathed in open natural water sources and as other primates do, they helped to keep one another free of bugs and debris. Trees and other sources of shade worked as sun-blocks, literally, and if shade couldn't be utilized when the sun was too intense, they smeared mud, clay, and wore some sort of clothing to cover sensitive areas from the sun. Sanitation in the form of bug removal, licking, spitting, and the use of plants to sterilize wounds dates back thousands of years. Hunter-gatherer groups today still use these methods to limit infections.

The living conditions of pre-agricultural humas were open and unsuitable for excess molds and mycotoxins. They moved about the land in a nomadic manner, never fouling or over hunting any specific location. They feasted and they fasted. They ate their food fresh and in season. They lived in their environment, bathed & cleansed in their environment, ate their environment, were eaten by their environment, they were an attributing part of their environment. They lived in sunshine, ate in the sunshine, admired, and even prayed to the sun and moon. They moved constantly as humans are designed to, walking, lunging, twisting, climbing, sprinting, dragging, pushing, throwing, creating etc.

These communities of early hominin followed large game through migrations and thus were often on the move, never settling in one specific area for very long. This part is essential to understanding the modern sanitation crisis. Before the farming revolution humans were free to move about the earth as they pleased. Once seeds were sown for the first time it meant that people had to stay nearby to defend and nourish their seeds for harvest. This led to larger and larger groups of people living in proximity, people acquiring and hoarding materials and thus power. As wild animals, the human population increased very slow. As agriculture improved, so did civilization, and craftmanship (out of necessity). This allowed the human population to explode. The transition from hunting and gathering to farming may have been created out of necessity, not out of choice. Many environments and climates around the world were changing and food was becoming scarcer.

At this point it became important to bring some of the game we used to hunt, into our living environment and make them "docile" or herdable at least. Sheep, goats, bovine, horses, hogs, chickens, ducks, and other small breeds became farm animals and pets. Living in close quarters with them, the now non-natural giant fields of mono-cropped plant foods and the pests that come with that led to new viral hopping issues. On top of this mess, since people weren't just leaving piles of fertilizer as they moved freely around the earth they were now growing in population and not moving, their bowels still needed expelled, but where to do it? This was and still is an issue in many civilizations. The need for specific places to put waste separate from the main water supply was important, this itself was one of the first forms of sanitization. Separating the waste from the water supply ensuring that the water sources were as clean as possible. Prior to this, humans needed little water, just enough to wet their lips occasionally but there was no need for the excess water it takes to water crops.

From this first sanitation onward there have been great leaps forward in keeping humanity safe and free from epidemics. But from the beginning of the farming revolution until about 5,000 years ago there isn't much evidence of epidemics plaguing humanity at all. There is though plenty of evidence of diseases sprouting up all over where man was eating lots of inconsistent foods to our biology. Throwing off our natural karma and destroying the earth all at the same time. Did you know that the desert where Egypt now stands was once an area of great abundance? The Nile River provided food and nutrients for many game animals and plant life. That's why they settled there. There was abundant water and life surrounding the civilization and it lasted for thousands of years until they slowly destroyed it through excessive farming. The Egyptians were some of the first humans (mostly upper-class Egyptians) to leave evidence of obesity and arterial disease. Even one Greek philosopher stated the prevalence of a sweet-smelling urine in patients (now we know that smell is from high blood sugar and is related to diabetes) that were overweight and sedentary. But still these people did not experience the immense society crushing plagues of modern history and cancer was still a rarity.

Consider that in 1950 some 75 million people lived in cities and now over 4 billion people live in cities. That is a lot of people living in proximity with little contact to nature and sunshine, simultaneously exposed to massive amounts of pollution (including EMFs).

The extreme reduction of individual human health and the weakened immunities of our communities led to these epidemics. Viruses have been around longer than humanity has, (1.5 billion years) meaning that we evolved with and around them. 8% of the human genome comes from viruses. Most viruses can only seriously hurt you if you have a weakened immune system or an immune system that has never encountered anything like it, like the Native Americans and the smallpox virus. The origin of smallpox is uncertain but some mummies from Egypt show rashes from the virus so it's likely that it had moved its way across Africa north to Spain and Northwestern Europe. The natural movement of the virus slowly across populations allowed for adequate time for peoples encountering it to build a bit of an immunity (even during a decline in healthy living conditions for most populations) before it found its way onto ships and sailed the ocean to a world with a population that had been far removed from where that virus had begun its progression through humans. We weaken our immunity to a point of easy access for these "bugs" by removing ourselves from the face-face community, eating garbage, inactivity, over sanitation, no fresh air, avoidance of sunlight, and stress. Amongst other things. Our current crisis is that of a collectively unhealthy population. Some research pertaining to the Spanish flu and the weakened immune systems of the world's population after the use of mustard gas and the polio epidemic after the use of heavily chlorinated community swimming pools in the United States will truly open your eyes. The underlying cause is never as simple as we have been led to believe. There is an even darker side to many of the recent "outbreaks" than just innocent people dying.

These catastrophes led to innovations in the world of cleanliness and sanitation meant to prevent and control them. At the time of these innovations and even now many people believed that they were the solution. Many, not knowing what the true problem was in the first place. It doesn't help that today, the sellers of said innovations do so in a way that make you believe you need them. Among these early novelties was bathing and washing. In the conditions humans were living in, this was probably a very pleasing practice to the nostrils. But they weren't doing it daily, or even weekly in most cases and they surely weren't using synthetically created fragrances and chemicals to clean their bodies under hot water that was treated with chlorine and fluoride. They went to a natural body of water and may or not have used soap at all, most of the soaps that were being used were made purely from animal fats, plant oils, pot ash, water, and or roots, you know, natural stuff. The kind that you will pay big money for today compared to the average bar of harmful suds.

As running water became more accessible, more frequent bathing became a cultural aspect that was attainable for more people. Prior to this, bathing was mostly revered as a spiritual and ritual practice. Humans would still of course do the type of "cleaning" or grooming that we observe in other animals, the picking, scraping, and scrubbing with or with-out a water source. As civilization grew and developed so did cleanliness practices. Ancient Egyptians would dress as Gods and bathe the dead ritualistically to assist in the transition to the afterlife. The Hebrews made laws regarding hand washing before and after eating and washing your hands and feet before entering a temple. Cleanliness could be closer to Godliness in many ritualistic ways showing respect and decency to the God(s). The Celts would use "clooties" (cuts of cloth) drenched in spring water to wash away illness from an individual, then the soaked cloth would be hung from a Hawthorn tree. The belief was that the cloth would absorb the energy that was making the person ill, and the Hawthorn tree would then remove that negative energy from the cloth so that it may be used again. Many sects around the world had similar beliefs regarding bathing and their respect towards natural water sources. As populations grew the necessity for a simplistic cleanliness practice grew, probably why the Hebrews made strict laws regarding this, especially prior to eating.

The history of soap

Hippocrates, a Greek physician prescribed bathing to cure many ailments, his ideas though had little to do with cleanliness. For him it was meant to balance the humors through hot and cold-water immersion, curing physical ailments like headaches and joint pain. Maybe this is why I feel so damn good after doing a hot/cold contrast hormesis session. The idea of this water immersion was more of a health-oriented practice than a communal practice but as the idea spread to Rome it became a leisurely and communal practice. As the Romans practiced this bathing, they introduced a sickle shaped device to scrape off mud and grime and would use plant oils. Some bathing practices though were not for self enhancement, the Aztecs bathed slaves before ritual sacrifices. Adversely in many cultures and religions it was frowned upon to bathe abundantly. As Saint Jerome stated, "He that is once washed in Christ needeth not wash again." And as Jesus himself proclaimed as he cautioned people for putting a religious ceremony over their inner purity "Cleanse first that which is within the cup and platter, that the outside of them may be clean also." Bathing was therapeutic, cultural, ritual, and spiritual. A much different practice than what we see today.

According to Roman legend, soap was named after Mount Sapo, an ancient animal sacrificing site. Rain washed the fat and ash that was leftover at the ceremonial alters down to the banks of the Tiber River. Women that washed their clothes in certain parts of the river noticed that after heavy rain falls their clothes were much cleaner. I don't know if this is the true origin, no one really does but it sounds good. We do know for sure that soaps themselves date back to at least 2800 BC in Mesopotamia where they used fat, water, and ash to create cylindrical shaped tubes of soap. A recipe was found written on a clay tablet and credited to the ancient Babylonians. If it was officially written in 2800 BC, you can bet that it was being made long before that. A scroll found in Egypt dating back to 1550 BC indicates the use of a similar soap using oils, wood ash, and water. A small soap factory was even uncovered in the remains of Pompeii, Rome which was destroyed by the eruption of a volcano in 79 AD.

Fast forward a few thousand years and people are slathering soaps (by that name, but not recipe) into each pore head to toe. To sell people on the use of soaps and bathing products entrepreneurs would have to convince the world that bathing with soaps was necessary for beauty, survival, and social acceptance. As the agricultural revolution progressed and people got sicker; bathing seemed to offer a solution to the growing number of environmental pathogens that humans couldn't eradicate. Still though at this point bathing was not a profitable business. Most families made their own soaps from fats/oils, water, and ash. Things that most families at that time literally had laying around. They would scent it with plants and plant oils if they were the luxurious type. Entrepreneurs looking to profit from the sale of soap had to compete with basically every homesteader and the market was still relatively small. By the early 1900's city people in the United States and elsewhere had begun taking weekly baths, they would fill a tub or basin with warm water heated by wood stove and bathe the whole family. This was quite the chore, but with the grotesque city living circumstances this weekly rinse was necessary. It's said that the last bath went to the youngest in the house, cold and filled with everyone else's grime and grease. Yuck! Although, it would have been a great immune booster.

As large-scale soap selling operations hit the road full throttle the first stop was at the mansions of the rich and royals. The higher classes have an excess of money and are often looking to make statements. A scented soap with a higher price tag and fancy name would help separate them even more from the regular folk. Royalty had already been using perfumes so the thought of being able to smell even better and be even cleaner and prestigious than the peasants put the cherry on top.

Since ritualistic bathing was the precursor to modern lathering, it makes sense that soap companies would initially utilize this type of advertising. By the late 1800's a few large corporations had already weaseled their way in the homes of innocent people just following the ads. Companies and entrepreneurs like Wrigley (yes, the chewing gum company), Proctor and Gamble, Colgate and Company, James Kirk, Nathaniel Kellogg Fairbank, and James and William Lever were plotting their way into every Americans bathtub. Ivory brand soap took directly from Psalm 45:8 "All thy garments smell of myrrh, and aloes, and cassia, out of the ivory palaces whereby they have made thee glad." After a bible reading at church William Proctors son Harley had the grand idea to name a new soap "Ivory". People at that time were well versed in the scripture so the bible did the selling for them once the name compelled them.

Palm Olive would eventually use the Queen/Goddess Cleopatra as a mascot. Cleopatra was not ethnically an Egyptian yet ruled as queen in Egypt and was known to be a living Goddess. She is often known as a Greek because this is where she traced her lineage. She was known for her beauty and apparently young and forever supple skin. Cleopatra bathed regularly in donkey milk and claimed this to be her secret of beauty. Palmolive contained no milk at all yet saw Cleopatra as the perfect symbol to sell their soap. And so, a marketing campaign utilizing her image on their palm and olive oil-based soaps began and consumers fell for yet another scheme. In 1906 Proctor and Gamble published a false yet believable advertising booklet titled "How to Bring Up a Baby: A Hand-Book for Mothers". Proctor and Gamble offered advice from a supposedly respectable and knowledgeable nurse on how to raise a baby and of course how to bathe them using their brands own Ivory soap.

The ad campaigns go on and on getting nastier and less true as time progressed. More companies hit the market with "new" soaps and new ads all the time, competition led to dirty ads. Literally. The use of black children in ads getting "lathered" to white and ads about keeping the cleanliness of a race, sexually transmitted diseases being caused by lack of cleanliness etc. As the times began to slowly but finally change in the 1930s' those ads started to go away, or at least be less obvious to the consumer. Large soap manufacturers still needed to convince people to buy soap, branding their soaps for even more specific uses and users gained traction. Suddenly soap with identical ingredients could be just for "Fido" or just for women's nether regions. Soaps for your kids, for Dad and for Mom, for your clothing and one for your dishes. There was a soap for everyone and everything. All being made from the same ingredients and many in the same exact factories.

Radio shows so-called *Soap* Operas hit the scene in the 1920s directly targeting home-making mothers and convincing them through very specific advertising that they needed to purchase soap. In the late 1940s and early 1950s Soap Operas hit the TV screen with the same intent as previously. Proctor and Gamble, one of the worlds' largest companies was the first to create soap operas and held on until 2009 when CBS announced that "As the World Turns" would be canceled, the last of the soap operas owned by the company. I was going to include a list here showing all the different companies that Proctor and Gamble owns but the list is far too extensive, instead I inserted a link to the SECs web page showing all the different companies that they own as subsidiaries and from there you can research all the products that they sell. Many isles in many stores, although looking like there are a variety of companies selling you specially formulated and "different" products, you'll find are all owned by the same people. https://www.sec.gov/Archives/edgar/data/80424/0001193125101 88769/dex21.htm

The first soaps were made from products that supported the skin microbiome and could have been eaten or even used to cook with, without causing harm to the consumer. These new age soaps were (and still are) made in factories out of substances that are not digestible, they strip the oils away from the skin without replacing them. Detergents, scents, solvents, sanitizers, and preservatives in these soaps wreak havoc on the skin microbiome and the havoc goes deeper, as these chemicals get absorbed into the skin and into the bloodstream, some of them even crossing the blood-brain barrier. Micro-plastics have been shown to make their way into the brain via the bloodstream.

In the mid to late 1800's it was presented that unclean hands were transmitting illness and thus the birth of everyday sanitizers. It was found that Alcohol efficiently sanitized germs from doctors' hands, stopping the spread of many deadly pathogens. This sanitation killed all the germs, good and bad. Billions of bacteria per square centimeter of skin on the human hand, most of which participate in the function of our immune system. Killing them is like having millions of troops placed all around an enemy, with a very heavy advantage and then right before you attack your enemy, you drop bombs all over your own troops. And then wonder why you keep losing these battles. Doesn't make much sense, does it? I am not arguing against sanitation in hospitals and during surgical operations, this is necessary. For regular people doing regular things, you should stay far away from hand sanitizers. Rinsing and cleaning off anything excessive that could be dangerous is a no-brainer but avoid anti-bacterial soaps and sanitizers unless it is truly necessary. Like, if you are about to perform open heart surgery.

I haven't showered, not like most Americans do anyhow for about three years now. I don't use shampoo, body washes, conditioners, deodorants, artificial fragrances or exfoliants under hot, treated water. I do rinse off my body and use a dry brush with a couple drops of organic essential oils soaked into the bristles when I feel the need (much less frequently than my previous 2-3 showers per day). I wash my hands when they are dirty, with a soap made from regenerative animal fats. I could lie and say that I do this because the average American shower uses roughly 20 gallons of fresh, perfectly potable water and the cleaning products used are filled with microplastics, chemicals, and ingredients that exploit and destroy ecosystems and people's lives in third world countries and destroy ecosystems and freshwater systems locally. But this honorable approach to a holistic and sustainable cleanliness routine isn't why I started.

For me it was skin complications. I was almost 30 years old and still dealing with teenage like explosive acne. At this point I had already begun changing my diet, attitude, and was exercising regularly, using sauna and cold plunges. It had gotten a lot more manageable but hadn't gone away. Prior to those changes I tried what was advertised to me. The acne seemed to get worse with each new product I tried. And I tried A LOT of different cleaning solutions and *cures,* but they all just seemed to dry out my skin long enough for a breakout to disappear and then come back with a vengeance. Leaving me scarred like I'd been in a fire. I was lost in the consumer search for a cure and was having a difficult time. My skin was seemingly becoming addicted to moisturizer, and I was slowly making the problem worse. I stumbled across some articles and research that glorified the sun and the skins natural microbiome for reversing cystic acne. I remembered back to when I was in my mid-twenties and experienced clear tan skin for about a year utilizing the sun, so I tried it again. Turns out, for me at least sun gazing and cutting out these harmful bath products were the final pieces to the puzzle. It didn't happen overnight, but it did happen quite quickly. I still encounter a pimple here and there, more frequently around the holidays when I may splurge for some of the sweet treats, alcohol, and dairy. Processed sugar and dairy (even raw), are my biggest *inflamers* so I avoid them as much as possible.

This was legitimately an issue I had been dealing with since I was an early teenager. At many points in my life, I

172

thought it would never change. I had even begun to except the fact that it wasn't going to change. I know now why the use of these products can cause irritation rather than fix it, you strip your skins natural protective oils and microbiome away with soaps and shampoos and then you replace them with harmful moisturizers. These products and practices are constantly throwing off your skins natural ecosystem allowing invasive species to reign supreme, causing micro-ecological imbalances.

Not using deodorant was a lot better than it sounds too. Honestly. At first, I noticed that pimples or sores that would sometimes plague my armpits disappeared, and I began to smell better, naturally. Since I had a good diet already, I didn't really stink. Even while breaking sweats daily at work, in the gym, and sauna. I do dip into a cold tub for a few minutes most days and after most sauna sessions too so that probably helps but it's nothing but a rinse off. Deodorants are filled with hormone disrupting chemicals and they block your pores in your armpit from doing their job. On special occasions I will slap on some deodorant. In the last two years I have gone through just 1 stick of deodorant. Its easier to find a good deodorant than you might think, treat that search like you do with typical body soaps.

As a mild disclaimer, fix your diet before expecting your skin to heal itself in this holistic approach. Utilize the sun and when you feel the need to rinse off do so. Use soap where you feel like you need to, just use good soap made with as few ingredients necessary. Don't shower under hot water, go out and get a filter for your shower head, one that filters out as many chemicals and toxins as you can find. I personally drybrush three to five times a week before using the sauna but you can do this before you take a shower or ice plunge as well, and this will dramatically increase the smoothness of your skin and help with scarring which is something that I'm working on now. Your skin replaces about 40,000 cells per minute throughout our entire lives, it is very efficient at replacing skin cells but don't over exfoliate, you don't want to exceed your skins capabilities. If you're going to use a dry brush like I do, I suggest analyzing your skin and listening to your body, do it lightly because you can cause a scratches and micro-abrasions.

Since removing crappy synthetic chemicals my skin has balanced out and now, I'm working on reducing the deep scarring from years of unhealthy skin. Initially I was in disbelief about the quick improvement of my skin due to not cleaning it. Since I had lived my entire life previously believing that I had acne simply because my skin wasn't clean enough. Weird concept when you think about it right? The human body is incredibly adaptable and a great communicator when things are not optimal.

My skin was telling me something was wrong through inflammation, but I wasn't receiving the message. The cause of acne in adults and teenagers alike have almost everything to do with hormone imbalances. We live in a world where basically everyone's' hormones are out of whack due to processed sugars, ancestrally inconsistent diet and lifestyle, microplastics, mycotoxins, lack of sunshine, water pollution, air pollution, heavy metals from foods/vaccines/pharmaceuticals, prescription drugs, illegal drugs, heavily treated water, being ungrounded from mother earth, emotional baggage, modern stresses induced by media and culture, lack of sleep, excess blue light and EMFs etc. The problem is worsened by the cleanliness industry and their sebum stripping agents and artificial moisturizers that decimate our skin microbiome.

Our skin replaces roughly 57,600,000 cells per day. that means we shed a whole layer of outer skin every two to four weeks, about nine pounds of skin cells per year. Our skin produces an oil called sebum to protect and moisturize it. Soaps can scrape and scar our skin, and when used daily the damage is too quick for our skin to properly heal. Many modern soaps strip off the oil that's there to protect it and maintain a healthy environment for our skin microbiome, this seems to trigger a reaction to produce more sebum creating a cycle of stripping and soaking. Our skin is our largest organ, if you're reading this book, you probably know that. If that's common knowledge, why do we smear toxic chemicals all over it? Would you scrub a toxic chemical all over your brain if it was exposed? Or all over your liver because some commercial told you that you needed to? That's essentially what we do today.

Our skin consists of three anatomical layers, the outermost is the epidermis. It's about a millimeter thick, about the thickness of a credit card. The keratinocyte is the primary cell of this outer layer, and they make the keratin protein that makes up most of our skin and the entirety of our fingernails and hair. There is a collage of immune cells and nerve fibers in this epidermis. The melanocytes are there as well. They react to our environment 24/7. It is separated into layers called strata that are determined by the age of the cells. The epidermis is constantly reproducing itself, faster than any other part of the human body. The basal layer of the strata is loaded with stem cells pushing up and replacing the outer most layer as the skin sheds. The cycle takes about a month. The nature of the outside world has determined this adaptation in human skin, prior to modern living this was plenty fast enough to maintain healthy skin.

The next layer is called the dermis. It is made up primarily of the two protein's collagen and elastin. This layer serves to give our skin elasticity and strength. Leather used for shoes, belts, wallets etc. is pure dermis because of its durability. The networks of nerves of these outer two layers can detect the slightest changes to our environment. A tiny spider on our neck or when the thermostat at home is a few degrees colder than normal. Follicles in these layers produce our hair. The skin needs sun light for proper health but also requires protection from excessive exposure. The skin is very complex, this complicated organ contains three types of glands that secrete oil and other compounds. The eccrine glands are the basic sweat glands. They secrete water to cool our bodies. The sebatious glands secrete sebum to moisturize and protect our skin. The apocrine glands are the ones we try to block with antiperspirants, deodorants, and fragrances, they are in our armpits and groins. All these glands sustain the microbes that live in and on us. Do your best not to inhibit their function.

Balding is Not the New Sexy

I don't care who told you that Dad bods and hair loss were sexy, it isn't true. My hair had started to thin out rapidly and I was starting to think I'd be a bald 35-year-old. I was thinking I could rock the Mr. Clean look. But, since removing shampoo, conditioner and consistently exposing my head to direct sunshine as often as I can, my hair doesn't appear to be thinning any more. I dry brush my scalp as often as I do the rest of my body and things are looking good. I can't say that it's thickening out and I now have long, thick, flowy locks but I am not continuing to go bald.

As general; holistic skin care advice, don't scrub down with plastic laden exfoliates, don't soak your skin with hormone disrupting chemicals, don't moisturize your skin with harmful substances and don't inhibit your ability to detoxify your body by sealing off your pores with anti-perspirants. Awakening the Tranquil Warrior with-in you is going to take coherence and health inside and out (skin/hair), top to bottom. Rinse off as often as you feel like you need to, cleaning the parts of you that sweat the most (creases, pits, and private regions) if you feel like you need soap then make sure you are using all-natural soaps void of chemicals. I recommend a soap made from fats; we prefer a tallow-based soap with essential oils as the fragrance in our home, but this is obviously your preference. Turn down the temperature in your shower, when you use scorching hot water, you are damaging your micro-warriors and drying out your skin. Try a cold shower, the health benefits are virtually endless, and your microbiome won't be negatively impacted. You'll even save money since you won't be heating so much water, and probably won't be in the shower as long thus saving money on water. Not to mention the minimalist fact that you will be wasting less water and using natural, biodegradable soaps that will not pollute our planet. Boom now you're playing your part.

Those Pearly Whites

You do everything the dentist tells you to, you brush, you rinse, you floss, you rinse again, you get your teeth scraped and cleaned by a professional twice a year, and yet your breath still stinks, cavities are still forming, and your teeth are yellow and deteriorating! How is this possible? While all the practices listed above may help slow the deterioration of your teeth, they do not prevent it and depending on the products you are using, they might be contributing to the break-down. In fact, fluoride (although hailed for its dental health benefits) disrupts your hormones contributing to insulin resistance, diabetes, and obesity. The standard American diet mixed with standard American dental care is a duo of dental destruction. Hormonal imbalances inhibit the body's ability to absorb and utilize minerals. Leading to weak teeth and bones.

Fluoride, touted as a savior for dental care, damages the pineal gland. Which secretes melatonin and is the primary source of the hormone. The pineal gland controls the sleep-wake cycle, and a lack of melatonin has been linked to a wide assortment of disorders like the obvious sleeping ailments that increase inflammation, weight management issues, and stress leading to high blood pressure, heart arrythmia, and of course cancer. Heart disease is the United States biggest enemy as it claims over 23% of all the deaths per year and Cancers claim additionally almost 22%. Melatonin deficiency has also been linked to neurodegenerative disorders like Alzheimer's disease. If you drink and bathe in fluorinated water, use a fluorinated toothpaste, rinse, and floss you may want to stop immediately. Each of the ailments listed above will decrease your body's ability to absorb minerals and nutrients meaning that your teeth will suffer. If your dental health is suffering, some other part of you is too.

Triclosan is another typical ingredient, it is a pesticide added to most toothpastes (and soaps). Triclosan is known to disrupt endocrine and immune function as well as irritate skin. Propylene glycol is added to many cosmetics including toothpaste as a softener. It is the main active ingredient in anti-freeze and has been linked to central nervous system damage. Paraben is also added to many toothpastes to keep them fresh longer and is one harmful chemical that we should all know by now as it has been removed from many utensils and food storage containers because of its known negative effects on the endocrine system, links to breast cancer, reproductive problems, and allergic reactions. The list of harmful additives continues and most of them have one thing in common. They disrupt the endocrine system. Why is this important concerning dental health?

The endocrine system regulates all biological processes in the human body. The system is comprised of multiple glands located throughout the body that release and receive hormones into and from the bloodstream and surrounding cells. Hormones act as chemical/electrical messengers controlling biological processes such as blood sugar control, growth (of everything), metabolism, reproductive health, appetite, and the survival fight, flight, freeze, or faint responses. The glands that make up the system from top to bottom are the pineal, hypothalamus, pituitary, thyroid, parathyroid, thymus, pancreas, adrenal, ovary (female), testicle (male), and placenta (pregnant female). The hypothalamus is the driver of the endocrine system and links the endocrine system to the nervous system. Hormone levels in your body are directly linked to your inflammatory response to infections and disease. Therefore, some women can experience what's known as pregnancy gingivitis. As you know during modern pregnancy hormone levels can become imbalanced leading to swollen and easily damaged gums that are more vulnerable to infection and gingivitis. Men and women alike with low testosterone experience higher rates of gum disease, heart disease, diabetes, and osteoporosis. People with thyroid disorders experience many metabolic issues but also dental health issues like gum disease, dry mouth, and a poor sense of taste. To fix your teeth, fix your hormones.

Poor dentin health is a pre-cursor to most infections of the tooth. Dentin is the hard-dense bone tissue that makes up the bulk of a tooth, beneath the enamel. Made of about 90% calcium and phosphorus (Howard University). Healthy dentin supports tooth structure, makes the enamel stronger, and prevents inner tooth infections and cavities from forming. Any negative disturbance in the way that calcium and phosphorus are metabolized and transported to the teeth and bones effects dental health. The endocrine system regulates all biological processes, this includes the maintenance of calcium and phosphorus homeostasis. Parathyroid hormone performs this duty. Inadequate intake of bioavailable calcium and phosphorus leads to the extraction of those minerals from the bones and teeth to provide support to other parts of the human body. Just as a pregnant woman's biological intelligence will take over and strip her own body of nutrients and minerals to ensure the health and wellbeing of her baby if she is not consuming enough nutrients and minerals. The human body is designed to survive, at whatever cost. We know that in a deep starvation mode our bodies will break down its own organs as fuel before we die, but most people don't realize that this process happens daily. Although on smaller scales.

Vitamin D's role in dental health is similar to its role in overall health. You need it. Calcium and vitamin D work hand in hand to maintain a healthy mouth. Your dentin contains little warrior cells that reside at the border of the enamel. These little border patrol warriors can repair damaged dentin. But only if you have adequate levels of vitamin D, if you do not, then your dentin defense system cannot perform its job.

When your nutritional and mineral intake is inadequate, your body will do its best to make up the difference. Even if it must break down your teeth and dentin to provide minerals to the rest of your body. The bottom line here is this, if you wish to keep all your adult teeth, keep them strong and healthy, then you must consume foods with adequate amounts of bioavailable minerals and nutrients, and spend adequate time in sunshine. As we age our absorption efficiency declines, which means our intake and the quality there of should increase.

The most important nutrients and minerals that you need for proper dental health are vitamin D, calcium, phosphorus, magnesium, vitamin A, vitamin K, and potassium. Increase vitamin D by exposing your skin to the sun and consume more organ meats, eggs, fatty fish, and grass-fed and finished ruminant meat. Utilizing the sun will always be the best way to increase vitamin D. Bone broth and bone marrow are great sources of bioavailable calcium and minerals. Liver is the single best source of vitamin A. Eggs; muscle meats and organs alike contain high amounts of bioavailable phosphorus as well. Fish, liver, meat, and eggs contain high amounts of bioavailable vitamin K, potassium, and magnesium all of which play a role in dental and bone health. (For the dudes out there, adequate amounts of vitamin D and K don't just make your teeth hard, they keep something else hard too, and one study states that the combo also increases the size of your package.) That should be enough for any man, or woman to make their man start eating raw liver, eggs, and bone marrow ¾ naked in the sunshine every day.

The products that we use in our mouth are particularly harmful because even if we do not swallow any of them, they get into our bloodstream and disrupt the function of our endocrine system. If your gums bleed when you brush, then these chemicals are getting there even faster. Dental health is directly linked to the individual's diet. Periodontal disease (severe gum disease) affects almost 9% of our population but it affects almost 22% of the diabetic population. To word it another way, less than a tenth of the average population has gum disease conversely a quarter of the diabetic population has gum disease. The effects that processed sugar and foods have on the endocrine system cause a multitude of disorders throughout the entire body and this includes your mouth. The food and hygiene additives we absorb daily only intensify the problem.

Early humans enjoyed much better dental health than we do today. They brushed their teeth while scraping meat off bones, flossed while pulling fat, tendons, and ligaments from between their teeth, and rinsed with the occasional gulp of water. Yet they experienced little dental decay compared to modern humans. The toothbrush we know as such today was invented in 1938, however evidence from ancient civilizations dates the novelty to 3000 BC. Chew sticks as they have been so logically coined were thin twigs with frayed ends that ancient peoples used to rub their teeth clean. As humanity began to eat more like ruminants with multiple stomach chambers and less like humans our teeth took a huge toll. The toothbrush became a necessary solution to a new problem.

Lack of minerals and essential vitamins leave teeth vulnerable to the effects of sugar. Both from sitting on the teeth and from the effects it has on the endocrine system. No worries though because once you restore your overall health your teeth can heal as well. For more specific information on this I highly recommend reading the book "Holistic Dental Care" by Nadine Artemis. As the shift in human diet from animal based to plant based and now to factory based continues the metabolic and hormonal effects are exasperating dental health.

69% of adults between 35 and 44 years old have lost at least one permanent tooth. As a country wide average by the age of 50, Americans have lost twelve permanent adult teeth and 26% of 65 to 74 years old have lost all their natural teeth. (Boston Magazine) The American Dental Association claims that 70% of Americans brush their teeth twice daily as recommended. Yet by 50 the average American has lost a dozen teeth? The CDC says that over 90% of Americans have had a cavity and that 1 in 4 Americans have untreated cavities. If you read anything else that CDC states, you'll read that fluoridation in water and toothpaste is to thank for Americans dental health. I don't know if "health" is the word I would use given the statistics listed above. Homo Erectus had a cavity rate of just 4.5%, while Homo Naledi and Neanderthals share a rate of roughly %1. Modern Americans have a cavity rate of 90%.

The differences in cavity rates between our ancestors and modern-day humans says a lot about the influence of diet and lifestyle on our dental health. High cavity rates are associated with heavy consumption of sugars, soft foods, and a lack of ruminant meat and tough foods that strengthen and nourish our teeth and jaw muscles. Eat like your early ancestors and you'll be able to chew with your own teeth until you die, at a ripe old healthy age. Since I switched to an ancestrally consistent diet, combining nose-tail nutrition with in-season, local, organic fruits, and some roots my gums have stopped bleeding while brushing, my teeth no longer hurt in the cold, and they are noticeably stronger.

While I don't think it's entirely necessary for our species to brush our teeth, I do believe teeth brushing was a great innovation in human evolution. Allowing us to eat a wider variety of food while maintaining somewhat decent oral care. Your oral care is essential for your longevity as many studies show that tooth decay and bad oral hygiene are precursors for early death.

Do your gums ever bleed when you brush your teeth? Mine used to. Whatever you are brushing your teeth with is going directly into your blood stream if they do. Fluoride, chloride, benzoate, potassium carbonate, micro-plastics and all those other destructive ingredients mentioned earlier are going straight to your blood stream. Your mouth is the first portion of the digestive system so what you brush your teeth with is getting digested even if you don't swallow. Another part of this issue is that most toothpastes are hard on your teeth. Silica and other ingredients are micro-scratching your teeth and tearing your gums apart each time you brush. Switch to a toothpaste with softer and less harmful substances. Since your mouth is stage one for digestion it's important to ensure the microbiome in there is prime to do its job efficiently. If they aren't prime, you aren't prime. Don't kill those little buddies with harmful chemicals.

My family enjoys Earth Paste brand, the chemical composition is satisfactory, still cleans your teeth and makes your breath smell great. You can also make your own toothpaste with some coconut oil, salt, or baking soda add a few drops of peppermint oil or spearmint oil to kick it up a notch. In the morning take a cup of salt-water and gargle and rinse for 30 seconds or so and spit it down the drain. This will help balance your mouths microbiome to keep away bad breath and promote healthy gums. Eating a diet void of processed sugar, and high in minerals will help even more.

Bathroom duties

Now, to the gross part of the bathroom sanitation system. Your bum. What are you using to clean after a healthy crap? Most people don't consider this a part of their holistic lifestyle regimen, but your butt has a direct line to the back end of your digestive track where all the blood vessels are for the absorption of nutrients. It absorbs what's there regardless of its way of entrance. Remember a few years back when college kids were getting alcohol poisoning from doing shots of alcohol down their keesters? They were dying and getting sick quickly because your body was not designed to handle or digest substances through this avenue. It *is* an exit after all. Our digestive system eliminates toxins, pathogens etc. and is meant to do so in one direction. Think about that next time you wipe with some cheap 2 ply in a supermarket bathroom. Whatever that paper is made from is going into your blood stream. I'm kind of a hippie about stuff like this so we use organic paper void of harmful chemicals. If you have one of those spray things that they use in other countries that's even better, I just recommend making sure it is filtered as well as you would your drinking water.

This goes for the ladies wiping their nether regions as well. If you are eating and living a well-balanced life you won't need to do any additional cleaning down there, it is a self-cleaning/self-balancing masterpiece that needs nothing extra from greedy corporations.

Sunscreens disrupt hormones

Let's leave the bathroom and head outside where we encounter another disruptor. Not technically a cleaner, sanitizer, moisturizer, or exfoliator but a skin product none-the less. I felt the need to address this one again. We covered its ability to efficiently block the glorious sun from gaining access into your cells, but we didn't fully discuss its destructive nature as it absorbs into our skin. Typical sunscreens contain many harmful ingredients like avobenzone that is known to break down quickly in the sun causing it to react more strongly with other ingredients, which in turn makes sunscreen manufacturers add other toxic "stabilizing" chemicals to the compound. Avobenzone is an endocrine disrupter and may be more toxic when exposed to chlorine, which of course is used in pools where children are often slathered in sunscreen. One of the chemicals used to stabilize avobenzone is octocrylene and it has been labeled a "possible carcinogen". Octocrylene breaks down into benzophenone which is a known hormone disruptor and a possible reproductive toxicant. Homosalate is another stabilizer added to sunscreens that has been found to be a "weak" endocrine disruptor along with a skin irritant but there is rising concern that it can accumulate in the body causing worse reactions in the future. Octinoxate has been banned by the state of Hawaii because it is a known reef killer. The Department of Health and Human Services (DHHS) determined that benzene (another popular ingredient in sunscreens) causes cancer in humans. Long-term exposure to high levels of benzene can even cause leukemia.

Not only does avoidance of the sun disrupt hormones but the chemicals in many sunscreens and lotions meant to keep the solar rays out of your body also disrupt them ten-fold. Avoid generic lotions at all costs, avoid sunglasses too they tell the most sensitive light receptors in your body that its dark out, and your body responds like it is dark, leaving your skin more vulnerable to sunburn and sun poisoning. If you need to use a sunscreen, choose one made with organic natural oils (not vegetable oils) and zinc as the main mineral blocker.

As of late there has been a lot of misinformation spread about SPFs and here's why. The sunscreen industry is worth roughly 10 billion dollars per year. If you follow the trail far enough you will see that most of the "different" sunscreen companies are owned by Johnson and Johnson. In fact, they own a lot of the "hygiene" products that Americans use today. 10 billion dollars is enough to pay a few people with some decent exposure to write a couple articles and call holistic practitioners quacks. And simultaneously promote the use of sunscreen. This is a sad but true reality, when it comes to profit vs health, big business chooses profit.

Us vs. germs, us vs. terrain, or us - is germs and terrain?

What is germ theory? In medicine, germ theory is the theory that certain diseases are caused by the invasion of the body by microorganisms that can consist of bacterial, viral, fungal, or protist species. The chemist and microbiologist Louis Pasteur (Pasteurization), surgeon Joseph Lister (Listerine), and physician Robert Koch are given much of the credit for development and acceptance of the theory.

What is terrain theory? Terrain theory states that **diseases are outcomes of our internal environment and its ability to maintain homeostasis against outside threats.** Terrain theory states if an individual maintains a healthy terrain, it can handle outside invaders that can cause diseases. When terrain is weak, it favors the invasive microorganisms. Basically speaking, germ theory states that any microorganism at any time can attack and wreak havoc on a human being, but terrain theory states that if one's terrain (immune system and body) is healthy, would-be attackers don't have a chance. We already know that when our grandparents said to "rub some dirt on it" or told our parents to "relax, the dirt is good for them" that they were right. Babies born vaginally get mommas microbiome, babies held by multiple people and exposed to animals and nature develop a much more efficient immune system than children born C section and sanitized daily. This is a fact. So why can't our culture admit it? If you have time and access to the inter webs right now I HIGHLY recommend going directly to this webpage https://www.westonaprice.org/health-topics/notes-from-yesteryear/germ-theory-versus-terrain-the-wrong-side-won-the-day/ and reading the article in its entirety. When you are done, come on back.

We evolved in out terrain, belong in our terrain, we *are* our terrain, we are about 40 trillion human cells that is carrying about 100 trillion microbes in and on us, so I think it's fair to say that we should look at immunity, like community and teach that we are germs, terrain, and us all at once.

Nutritional skin care specifically for women pre, during, and post pregnancy (Kate's Entry)

While I was pregnant with our first little one, I was afraid to get stretch marks, not just afraid, I was literally crying and terrified that my body would be *ruined*. (I know it's very superficial but being so young (21 years old), this was a devastating thought). I spent endless hours scouring the internet and reading everything I could on how to combat the appearance of or eliminate the chances of having stretch marks. I worked in the beauty industry as a cosmetologist for several years prior with interest in skin and hair, but I only knew one side of the story. The story of *you need to buy this, apply that, soak in this, smear this, clean with this,* the industry teaches us that we *need* some specially formulated, overpriced, and mass produced, product to have sexy skin. I came across many products from the store or salon skin brands that advised the user to apply twice a day, but on these products that where "safe" to use on my body there would be ingredients that I knew where not safe to consume, and I knew that my skin absorbed what I put on it, it also didn't make any sense to me that these products would hydrate the skin. I had the quick thought while in the supermarket aisle "If I need to apply this twice a day is this truly hydrating? Shouldn't once be enough?" second thought was "Wait, how is anything on this ingredient list like parabens, formaldehyde, triclosan, phthalates, etc., mixed with several types of alcohol, fragrances and color dyes good for my skin?"

Not only are those ingredients *not good for your skin,* but they are also dangerous. Consider this, in Europe today 1,328 chemical ingredients are banned from use in cosmetic products due to their potential risks, ranging from genetic mutations, reproductive health, endocrine health, and carcinogenesis. In the United States of America there are only 11 restricted chemicals in cosmetics. This is extremely concerning to me because I know so many girls around my age that are experiencing hormonal issues that they shouldn't be, so many young girls, blessed with the capability of creating life, are unable to do so.

Our skin is an organ, an organ that accounts for 16% of our body mass. An organ that absorbs everything that we slather onto it. A recent study by Statista found that 52% of U.S. consumers use skincare products daily, while just 6% reported not using any skincare products at all. This shows that 94% are using skincare products, and likely have absolutely no idea about the toxic chemicals in these products.

Learning all of this opened my mind to investigating what would truly work and changed the way I looked at skincare forever. Like most first time mothers, I was concerned for my health and of course my baby's health, I wanted to make sure I was giving us both everything we needed to be the healthiest expression we could be. My first pregnancy I used a mixture of shea butter and coconut oils applied after the shower, onto my belly, but I would still notice how dry my skin could be, so I dug a little deeper. I read that unrefined is better for the oil and I also swapped out for organic products assuming that some pesticides must obviously leak through your skin in the process, right? Turns out, my initial assumption was right, pesticides do get absorbed into your skin through skincare products. I did this and it did work to minimize the appearance of my stretch marks and improve the elasticity of my skin for both of my first two pregnancies (that were born just under 11 months apart).

By the time of my 3rd pregnancy, I had really drifted into the holistic study of the body and skin, I had become certified in holistic nutrition in 2017, fast forward to 2021 I gained true knowledge on this topic through experience and lots of additional research. Nutrition should be looked at as everything we consume, not just what we eat but what our skin consumes, what our energies consume, and what our mind consumes as well. *That* is holistic nutrition.

I stumbled upon a new field of research, the microbiome of the body and how everything you apply to your skin affects it. This was a groundbreaking thought for me, I had never thought of my skin as its own world full of flourishing life that loved to work together and was designed to. After several books and podcasts on the skin and gut connection I was able to connect what I had learned through holistic nutrition to deepen my holistic approach to skincare.

The gut microbiome houses much of our body's knowledge, what you consume physically and mentally directly affects your skin. It's your body's way of telling you of any internal problems that are going on, it's the outward communication that says "Hey! Over here! What you ate last night... yeah, we're not a fan of; would rather you not eat that k? thanks." Skin inflammation is a signal that something internally is not right, our skin naturally heals rapidly after damage but when the damage is occurring all the time, every mealtime, every time we get stressed out, or every time we encounter an allergen, we don't ever get to see our skins miraculous healing power.

We are stressed out and know that stress causes acne but why? Stress creates anxiety which stirs up all those tiny gut bacteria because our hormone levels are changing and sending signals and messages from the brain down our vagus nerve to our belly, and many more messages coming from our belly directly to the brain. Our body's give us ample signals and messages when we damage it, but we ignore these messages. We just carry on covering them up in chemicals, creams, foundations, facials, prescriptions that are not fixing the problem within our body's, they are literally just *covering them up, like cover up makeup,* and so the damage and inflammation just keep reoccurring and eventually worsen and turn into auto-immune diseases, we push off signs that our body is communicating to us so often that the body must find new ways to communicate it's dysbiosis, discomfort, disharmony, dis-ease. Over time these missed signals worsen and manifest into other dis-eases and larger symptoms than "just a zit" or minor inflammation.

Working Inward towards Outward (Kaitlyn Sweet)

Think of your body as one super system that is here FOR YOU not ever against you, it wants you to be abundant and to flourish, it will do everything in its power to make you that way. The body is the beautiful temple of the soul and creates a home where it can reside and enjoy all that the human experience has to offer. How beautiful is that?

How do we give our temple everything that it needs so that we can enjoy this human existence to the fullest? Eating good fats is one of the biggest secrets to maintaining a beautiful temple. Consuming good fats are essential for skin and stretch mark redemption! My 3rd pregnancy I did as holistic as I could. I fed my skin and its microbiome the things it needed to be happy. I let my skin get oily and just showered under the water purely with a tallow, elderberry soap bar or an olive oil, sage bar. Dry brushed my belly and whole body twice a week before showering sometimes in the sauna (I went no greater than 120* and 20 minutes while pregnant), consumed a good amount of homemade organic bone broths, bone marrows, tallows, lards, coconut oil and olive while cooking, consumed good amounts of smoked salmon and grass fed and finished liver, avocados, sometimes almond butter. Avoid cooking theses oils that are plant based like extra virgin olive oils at high temps because it can easily damage the oil contributing massively to inflammation, and cellular damage caused by oxidative stress. (Coconut oil can be used at a higher temp because it is a heat stable saturated fat.) Also look for the bottles or jars that are darker in color! Something not a lot of people think about is the darker colored bottle protecting that oil because these delicate fats can be damaged by excessive exposure to light. Always go for the glass bottle and not the plastic bottle of any oil you buy or any food product for that matter. Plastics can easily leak into the products.

Proteins play a role in your skincare as well; they are building blocks for human life. Each cell in the human body contains protein which require amino acids to build new cells. There are 20 standard amino acids with all having different functions in the body. Food contains a mix of protein sources; some contain all of them and some contain less of them. The ones that contain all protein sources are called "complete proteins" while others that contain a select amount are called "incomplete proteins". Foods of animal origin like eggs, dairy, fish and meat are complete proteins. Plant foods like beans, legumes, nuts and seeds are incomplete proteins. Eating a mix of both is a wise choice for overall skin health during pregnancy and not pregnancy.

Omega 3s otherwise known as DHAs are especially important here as well, not only do these fantastic fats play a huge role in brain and vision development in pregnancy it also is a great fat to be consumed for the body pre and post pregnancy. These fats will help nourish your skin from the inside out, helping to prevent and manage the stretch marks from pregnancy.

DHA is found in fatty fish (eat small breeds of fish, they contain much lower amounts of heavy metals), grass fed and finished beef, bison, deer, elk, and pasture-raised eggs. The Omega Fat you would want to avoid consuming large amounts of is Omega 6. Omega 6 is linked to a list of things such as abnormal brain development, increased risk of disease in fetal, and anxiety later in life when mothers consume too much while pregnant. Studies show that consuming too much omega 6 rich oils coming from corn, soy, cottonseed, canola, and safflower oil inhibits the synthesis of DHA, avoid vegetable oils at all costs. The oils listed above should never be consumed or smothered onto your largest organ.

Prioritize high quality animal foods whenever your budget will allow. The fats in animal products like meat, dairy, and eggs are directly affected by what those animals have been consuming themselves. Ruminant animals that have been grass fed and pasture raised are higher in Omega 3's and lower in Omega 6's, pasture raised eggs are also more nutritionally valuable compared to conventionally raised hens. Bonus! The flavor of grass-fed and pasture raised meats is so much better compared to animals that have been cooped up and force-fed soy and grains inconsistent with their ancestral diet. It will be an easy transition on the taste buds.

I wish I could say I have always eaten this way but only within the last 6 years have I made these changes and it has been a ROAD. Thankfully, Trenton and I traveled this road together, learning how to prepare and cook new foods in a multitude of ways, learning and teaching one another as we traversed the world of nutrition.

I was the type of child that ONLY consumed sugar and boxed snacks, pops, fast food, and little Debbie's. I even worked at fast food joints mostly in my teenage years, I thought it was gross then but still consumed it every day! My go to breakfast was without a doubt a honey bun from a vending machine or some form of a snack cake with a pop or energy drink.

Even at the beginning of our journey, as we reached out in programs and outside learning It was so much to consume and take in, so many differing opinions on topics like fats for example. Our society has been teaching us since we were little that fats are so bad for us, that they cause disease and make us fat. Especially saturated fats, they taught us were the worst. It took me forever to adjust my brain that eating and consuming saturated fat was what my body needed. I still remember when someone told me butter was good for brain development. At that time, I was learning that low fat diets were the way to go (NOT TRUE unless you were high amounts of fat from trans-fat laden vegetable oils and deep-fried foods. Then going to a low-fat diet will make you healthier, but just because your previous diet was trash.) I thought at that time "What?!" I was in disbelief of what they said I thought "You are straight crazy! Whoever told you that must have liked butter because that is a good way to get so fat you have trouble tying your own shoes." Here I am, proven completely wrong and in fact it has changed my life and how my body responds to work outs, sun light, brain health (brain fog), and skin health. My husband once told that he read Eskimos, and native Alaskans ancestrally consumed large amounts of animal fat; blubbers, like 99% of their diet was animal foods, very fatty animal foods that they even consumed mostly raw. Doing this gave them very healthy, elastic skin compared to other people, especially modern people, and women had much easier births, much easier recovery from birth, extremely low rates of birthing difficulties and their skin was amazing! When Trenton told me this I thought "That is wild", but truth is most ancestral humans ate in this way. Not only did they consume fatty animals' nose to tail, but they also used the leftover fats on the exterior of their bodies for bathing and lotions. They did not contain any of these fillers and by-products or fake scents that we use now. Completely naturally moisturizers and soaps, ones that if you try to buy from a health store can cost a fortune.

We live in a culture that provides very little truth about holistic nutrition, especially when it comes to skincare, pre-conception nutrition, prenatal, post-natal and breast-feeding nutrition and health care that many young women today are struggling with, it makes me sad to see this, and I hope that my addition to *Awakening the Tranquil Warrior* is helpful to you or any women you know! My final guidance on this topic is that if you cannot eat it, don't put it on your skin. If it has vegetable oils in it like the ones I mentioned before, don't eat it or use it on your skin.

My absolute two FAVORITE BOOKS of ALL TIME for learning about a true holistic pregnancy are "Real food for Pregnancy" by Lily Nichols and "The First Forty Days" by Heng Ou. These two books literally changed my life, and the lives of our children. Plus, there are some super delicious recipes in them! (Kaitlyn Sweet)

CHAPTER SIX

ENERGY

Imagine that you are in a dense crowd of people, downtown in a large city, standing elbow to elbow with thousands of people, people are bumping into you from all sides, between the chatter of thousands of people, cars bustling, horns honking, and loudspeaker advertisements you can barely hear yourself think. That image alone might induce some emotional reactions in your body. Maybe fear or excitement? For me it sparks a bit of anxiety. Now imagine that in that crowd you feel something strange, like a tug on your back pocket or your purse. You immediately check for your belongings and realize that you've been pick pocketed, as you scan the people around you, you realize that no one else noticed or cares, and the thief is long gone. Now maybe you're feeling anger, anxiety, or panic? Minor I'm sure since it's just an imagination exercise. Regardless, unless you are a sociopath you would feel a rush of chemically driven emotions in that real world event. Chemical/electrical reactions are the base of all emotions.

The word emotion has Latin roots in the form of 'emovere' meaning to move, move out or move through'. Emotion is the movement of energy out and through its starting place. Break down the word emotion to e-motion, the "e" standing for energy, making it energy in motion. Energy in the form of emotion moves electrically, chemically, and hormonally throughout and around your body. Good and bad emotions alike release chemicals that release hormones that make you feel a particular way. If you have spent a good part of your life feeling a certain way, good or bad, your body will crave that feeling. That feeling even if it's terrifying will remind you of who you are, it will provide you with a sense of control because you recognize the energy and have accepted its presence in your life. You will want to feel that contentment. Meaning you will find reasons to put certain energies in motion. People who were abused as children often endure abusive marriages and adult lives. Not because they *want to* but because these feelings have created deep and powerful neuropathways and at a certain point the body believes this is how their life is supposed to be.

To be the best version of yourself you will need to understand, manage, and utilize these energies in motion. Many of the habitual energies we drive into motion are damaging to us. To awaken the tranquil warrior inside of you, you will need to get to the core of your deepest traumas. Some may be from this lifetime, some may be from a previous one, some may have been passed down epigenetically from your parents or even ancestrally. You will have to dig deep, finding the blockages and traumas, resolving them, and letting them go. Developing new understandings of the innerworkings of yourself and others along the way.

Blockages in the flow of your vital life force will lessen the effects of everything else we have talked about in this book. You can eat ancestrally consistent, move in an ancestral manner, avoid toxins, poisons, processed sugar, EMFs, blue lights and spend adequate time grounded, under the sun and still not get exactly where you want to be physically, mentally, or spiritually. You will undoubtedly lose excess fat, increase muscle strength and function, increase cognitive function, decrease stress, increase physical capabilities, decrease negative excitability, increase mood, and limit, prevent, or even cure yourself from many other ailments. But to go that final step and really be the tranquil warrior that you are destined to be, you will need to master your own emotions. Mastering your emotions is no walk in the park, you've been warned, you will be fighting against millions of years of biology that want to cling on to these emotions as a survival mechanism, but you must overcome this primal behavior. Be primal in every other way of life, besides allowing the fight, flight, freeze, or faint responses to control you.

Thinking, meditating, breathing, energy clearing, and intense physical stress are my favorite ways to address trapped emotions and limiting beliefs. Thinking is the easiest so we can start there. "Your brain is a three-pound universe that processes 70,000 thoughts each day using 100 billion neurons that connect at more than 500 trillion points through synapses that travel 300 miles/hour." (Healthybrains.org). The better half of these thoughts are self-limiting and regressive for most people. Perpetuating the perception that the environment is dangerous. Thus, communicating to your cells that you are in constant danger, telling them to allocate all their resources to immediate survival while dismissing longevity. Whilst ancestrally this served to protect us from real threats, today its excess contributes to inflammation, disease, cardiovascular disease, and cancer.

Start utilizing your thoughts to improve your life. You have 70,000 chances to change the way you think. And that's just today! Become mindful of what you are saying to yourself, correct your thoughts when they are regressive or limiting. Replace self-limiting beliefs with a mantra that speaks to your current goals. For example, when you have noticed several limiting thoughts pass by in a short amount of time you can recite to yourself something like "I am love, I am loved, I am loving." Feel the power of each word in your mantra. Whatever you need to know and reassure yourself will differ situationally, don't be ashamed that you are talking to yourself. You literally do it 70,000 times per day anyways. They are YOUR thoughts; they should be helping you achieve your goals not diminish the results of your hard work.

My wife and I tell our kids that "the words you think and say are magic spells so be sure to cast good ones, and don't cast any that you don't want to come true." When you think and say anything, you are sending those vibrations; frequencies out into the universe, and the universe will respond in harmony. This is known as the law of attraction but can also be thought of as the quantum realms version of like likes like. Think of words and phrases like godspell or now gospel or even cursing someone using curse words. As simple as a word might be, when spoken it moves the atmosphere and literally vibrates from one person to another causing a sound that can be heard and perceived at a conscious sensory level, but they also carry a frequency in the form of emotion. Making spoken words more powerful than your thoughts. Be careful of what you say to people and yourself.

You send out 70,000 thoughts per day, 70,000 different signals to the universe that you are aligned in a certain direction. The universe will harmonize with that frequency, and you will continue down that path of thought, emotion, action, and reaction. Living the same day repeatedly if you can't change the way you think.

How to change the way you think. The English language that we speak today is directive and overly possessive. For example, we say, "I am sad" whereas in Irish you say that "sadness is upon me. Whenever you say that you *are* something you are making statements about a permanent reality. Conversely, when you say that you have sadness, or that sadness is upon you, it speaks to the temporary state of the emotion. Speaking this way out loud will surely make people look at you funny in the United States but the point is to understand the importance of the words you say out loud and inside your own head. Like they cast spells, because they do, you curse people with harmful words and raise them with praise. Don't say that you are sad, or mad say that you are feeling sadness, or madness, insinuating that those feelings will go away in due time.

It's the beginning of your work week and you are talking to a friend, and you say, "I *have* to go back to work". Change just one word in that sentence and the emotion changes entirely. "I *get* to go to work." Say those two sentences out loud and feel the difference in the energy just by changing one word. If thoughts are the language of the mind, then feelings are the language of the body. Choose your words wisely because they influence your feelings and the way in which your cells perceive the environment and at a quantum scale, this alone changes everything around you.

Have you ever felt the mood change mid conversation? Sometimes it happens when you say something you shouldn't have or maybe just something you said recollected a bad memory in someone or maybe you intimidated them or made them feel uncomfortable somehow. That is quantum energy moving in the form of emotion through everyone involved, because of a thought or feeling that someone had that shifted the frequency they were expressing, that shift extends far beyond just their body. As each cell perceives a *threat* or harmful emotion each cell responds defensively at the speed of light, reflecting their emotional energy onto the people around them.

Meditation

Meditation has become a bit of a buzz word around the health and wellness community and for good reason. Evidence of the immense benefits from meditation have been stacking up for thousands of years and with the advancement or neuroscience and quantum physics, the scientific proof is mounting quickly as well. Each of the 40 trillion or so cells that make up the human organism perceive the outer environment through signals that we provide. Chemically, electrically, hormonally etc. They react to this perception immediately, precisely, and unconsciously. The modern world, although not nearly as stressful as we perceive it, *is* still stressful. When we live in a way that we are looking for problems to worry about, our cells perceive the outer environment as dangerous, keeping their trigger fingers on the weapon of mass destruction/protection known as fear response. Breaking old habits like this is easier through meditation. If you have done everything else in the previous chapters and begun realigning your thoughts, then meditation will be a breeze. Just kidding, meditation is difficult, that's why it's called a practice. Your meditation practice will progress, and progress leads to less mess, stress, and better sex.

For every one minute of meditation, you gain 9 minutes of productivity, I found this out in a book I recently read called "How To Train Your Mind" by Chris Dailey. The author measured his amount of time of production without meditation and his amount of time of production with meditation and broke it down into a mathematical formula that he could better understand the gains he would have by adding a meditative practice. He found that the quieter you were able to make the mind for a longer period, the more production the mind would gain. He used a 30-minute example, 30 minutes of meditation daily produced 270 abundant minutes of productivity that he wouldn't have had otherwise.

No meditation explanation would be complete without mentioning the pineal gland. This gland produces melatonin (a precursor to DMT). Melatonin is an important hormone for reaching higher states of consciousness. The pineal gland was known to ancient cultures as the third eye and is depicted as such in many ancient texts. A few things that the tranquil warrior in you has already done, because nothing in this book should be taken for granted, have already improved the function of this gland. You should be sleeping better and remembering more dreams already. Removing fluoride and processed sugar, increasing exposure to natural sunlight, and reducing your exposure to EMFs will massively improve the function of this gland making meditation easier and more rewarding.

Meditating is one of the simplest ways to de-stress and heal. You don't need any special contraptions, chairs, music, essential oils, mind-altering "drugs" or even a professional meditator to guide you. These things can help you, but, ultimately, the quality of your meditation is on you. Ancient civilizations across the planet practiced meditation to connect to divine spirits for knowledge, guidance, protection, war tactics, hunting success, and rain for a better harvest. Civilizations small and large from across the entire planet used mind-altering substances to facilitate a much more vivid experience. Some practices used psychoactive plants and mushrooms to achieve higher more lucid states, some used extreme heat (saunas), extreme cold (ice plunging), extreme states of physical stress, or a combination of all the above.

All those additional "hacks" were used ceremonially with the guidance and support of their respected tribes with a specific goal in mind. This is not necessary. All you need is a safe and quiet place to sit or lay down. Somewhere that you will not be disturbed, and somewhere that if you fall asleep you will be safe. Dr. Joe Dispenza has completed many scientific studies on the bodies capacity to heal and rewire itself to create new ways of living. He recommends beginning your meditation in the early hours of the morning or late hours of the evening. During these times your natural levels of melatonin are higher, and you can achieve more transparent and meaningful states of consciousness. DMT, most notably heard about on Joe Rogan's podcast, is produced by the pineal gland and many people believe that through meditation, breathwork etc. that DMT levels can be increased enough to achieve a mind-altering experience. I have experienced my most influential and awakening meditations early in the morning when melatonin levels are the highest and the pineal gland is functioning optimally. I don't know if it's the dimethyltryptamine increase that allows me to transcend my physical body but, whatever it is, I like it.

Many people have and will continue to do ceremonies using concoctions like Ayahuasca to achieve a higher state of consciousness and to connect to the divine. Although, as I described in the introduction that I have used illegal drugs, I have never tried any of these ceremonial substances especially in that manner. When I learned of these rituals, I was providing for my family in a career that required monthly urine and hair samples to ensure I wasn't using illegal substances. As a father and husband, I take great pride in being able to provide for my family, I was unwilling to sacrifice my family's security for a moment of divine connection. Especially when I realized that I could achieve this state of consciousness without risking my career. I will sometimes put together a cocktail of legal substances like lion's mane mushroom powder, cacao, cayenne pepper, steamed coconut milk, coconut oil, cinnamon, nutmeg, cardamon, Celtic Sea salt, and sometimes turmeric powder and black pepper prior to breathwork, meditation, hot/cold contrast work, intense physical exercise, energy clearing/accepting, or any spiritual practice for that matter.

Noting here that historically high priests, shamans, witch doctors, and spiritual guides of all kinds used substances to achieve higher states of divinity. Early religious ceremonies included frankincense, myrrh, cinnamon, and cannabis, which in a fumigated mixture have hallucinogenic, opioid like effects, fumigated publicly for the people to enjoy and connect spiritually. Privately the high priest would basically hot box this concoction or one like it to get as close as possible to God and receive wisdom. Manna also known as *angel's food* or *bread of heaven*, later replaced with regular bread was "thin flakes like frost on the ground" (Exodus 16.14) described to taste like wafers made with honey, according to the Jewish treatise the Zohar, manna imparted sacred knowledge of the divine. The collaboration of fumigations, wine, and manna (fungus, insect secretion or something else, very sugary provided a dopamine rush) must've had early congregations truly one with God. The use of ayahuasca, psilocybin mushrooms, toad skin secretions and more were used around the world to facilitate greater connections to the almighty. The *Stoned Ape Theory* presented by Terence McKenna the author of "Food of The God's" theorizes that humans have been experimenting with psychoactive substances (mostly psylocibin mushrooms since we followed the herds of cattle that these mushrooms grow in), for tens of thousands of years, probably much longer. And this experimentation led to our higher state of consciousness through epigenetic evolution. As of today, I cannot vouch for any of these substances, and I recommend that anyone looking to use them find a very safe place to connect and a safe guide to assist you on the journey.

When you begin your meditation practice make sure that you empty your bowels and bladder so that you are not disturbed. Make sure that you will not be bothered by anyone or anything for a while, this includes pets. Give yourself extra time in case you achieve a great meditation. Trust me, you won't want to leave that space. Get into a comfortable position laying or sitting down, start by focusing your energy on an intention. Whatever you intend on manifesting into reality. Do you wish to heal from an auto-immune disorder? Do you wish to heal from past traumas? Do you wish to connect with your spirit guides? Whatever the intention may be just set it. I mean really set it. Be deliberate and believe in your intention. Once you've set your intention begin focusing on your breath, breathing in through your nose, filling your belly and lower chest. Releasing the breath comfortably out of your nose as well. If thoughts that do not match your intention start to flood your mind you need to acknowledge them, acknowledge their importance, and then let them go. Letting your mind know that you will get to those concerns later, you are safe, and in the middle of something much more important.

Another popular style of meditation that you probably already do a few times a week is called a moving meditation. Moving meditations are the easiest way to meditate, the easiest way to silence your mind because you are engaging in a physical task that you can focus on exclusively, like you do when you put all your attention on your breath. Only in a moving meditation you are placing all your attention on something more physical, which is much more entertaining for the mind, so it's easier to quiet it. Athletes refer to the feeling you get during a moving meditation as the *flow state*. And if you've ever been there, you won't want to leave. It is a blissful place where your entire being is working in harmony and everything is falling into its proper place miraculously with seemingly zero effort. You don't have to be an athlete though to engage in this flow, as the Pixar Film "Soul" plays out on the television screen, a flow state can be reached focusing, enjoying, and doing practically anything that you love. Writing, singing, playing instruments, dancing, fishing, walking, hiking, yoga, working on cars, swinging kettlebells, or anything else really.

Depending on your intention you will send your energy and attention to different places. If you are interested in connecting to a higher self then focus your attention on your third eye, pineal gland, top of your head (crown), or the space just a few inches above your head. Focus your attention, intention, and breath to this area. If you want to heal from something particular in your energy field, you will need to know what energy center that damage resides in. Focus your energy there. If you are intending to heal a wound or discomfort in or on your body, then focus your attention on that specific part of your body. If you wish to achieve a goal or manifest something into your physical reality, then focus there. It's that simple. Take as much time as you need, feeling the love, health, and vitality flowing through you. Feel the healing powers, feel the love, feel the divine flooding into you, truly feel the result of what you are intending. Throughout your meditation it is important to know, understand, and feel that you are one with everything and have the power to create anything you wish.

Meditation is a practice, meaning that some days you will perform very well, other days may be lackluster. But overall, you will see progress. Some days you will feel a burning desire to go meditate and others you will find it laborious. If you find yourself thinking of this practice as a chore, don't force it. The results will be less than desired. You can use some of the tools listed earlier if you feel like you need help calming down and getting into that head space more efficiently. I prefer scents and sounds. Lemon verbena, palo santo, patchouli, and nature sounds really get me "vibing". Working some kundalini style breathwork like breath of fire (quick inhales through the nose into the belly and quick exhales pulling the belly in), Wim Hof style breathwork, 30-40 deep breaths through the nose and into the belly, without a pause exhaling. Then a breath out and holding your breath for as long as you can, followed by a recovery deep inhale and hold. Repeating this for 3-5 rounds. If the mind is the gateway to higher states of consciousness, then breath is the transportation mechanism.

Breathing is free, and through working with your breath you can induce altered states of consciousness and emotional states. I prefer the style of meditation explained in the previous paragraphs, but the most common type of meditation is breathwork-based. It sounds easy, just focus on your breath for 2-30 minutes. Until you try it. Breathing is a function that we typically don't think about until we can't. When you bring your focus and attention on it you will realize how boring your breath really is, this will send your mind racing and gushing over random concerns and situations. We take an average of 22,000 breaths per day and are mindfully focused on very few of those breaths. I have begun to understand the breathwork style of meditation like this, if you can focus on your breath without distracting yourself, you can focus on *anything*. When you begin working with your breath during meditations it is much easier to breath in a specific way so that focusing on it becomes a task for the mind to accomplish, limiting the number of times it wanders. Kaitlyn and I are fans of the *Wim Hof Method* and most commonly choose that style of breathwork during meditations. I also enjoy box breathing, four second inhale, four second hold, four second exhale, four second hold and repeat for as long as you wish.

Open up buttercup, you've got work to do

Part of allowing yourself to be the tranquil warrior that the universe intended, means you must be open to new practices. You need to be willing to grow and let go simultaneously cultivating a new environment for the self that you wish to create while letting go of the self that you were or currently are. Ethan Suplee (Actor/Podcast Host) says about his epic weight loss, "I killed my clone". Give yourself the opportunity while letting go of who you were to reflect, respect, and acknowledge the, *you* that used to be. Then bury that *you* and use it as fertilizer to nourish the new *you* that is awakening.

I practiced yoga as a teenager and at the turn of my 20s but only because I thought it was helping me to be more flexible for the sake of athletic competition. I never thought of yoga as a spiritual practice. I now know that's exactly what yoga is. My wife began doing yoga at a fitness studio a few years ago and really loved it, she brought me to a few classes, and I enjoyed it as well, these were stretch and flow kind of sessions. Then, my wife had an awakening and decided that she wanted to become a yoga instructor, explore the spiritual side, and expand her knowledge.

She manifested the opportunity to study and become certified in yoga and found a little studio offering instructor training and signed up. She began practicing yoga there as well and introduced me to many spiritual practices that were previously outside of my wheelhouse. This place where she started her journey is a hole in the wall kind of studio, nothing fancy, nothing out of the ordinary. Until you meet the owner and the people that work in the studio. You can feel the energy when you walk in the door. Like that scene from Doctor Strange where he begins his spiritual enlightenment prior to acquiring his powers. This place is like nothing either of us had ever experienced. The studio is filled with compassion and there's an overwhelming feeling of protection and guidance. I am a natural skeptic, but I also know that deep down, if I want to experience something at its fullest then I must trust and respect the process. I know that I must surrender to the situation and let the energy flow as naturally as I can allow.

One day, as Kaitlyn and I had started to delve deeply into our spirituality she asks me if I would be willing to do this "Emotional Code" class that her new yoga teacher performed at the studio. I am not afraid to try new things so obviously I said yes. That night I researched what it was all about and thought, okay, this is a highly suggestive therapy. The practitioner walks you through some past *traumas* and unhealthy periods of your life giving you a vague time frame and then you go "Oh yeah, I did feel overwhelmed between the ages of 14-18." Then the practitioner releases that trapped emotion and you move on to another one. As the skeptic in me grew, I realized that I was ruining the experience for my wife and I before it even happened so I let it go and told myself that I would trust and surrender to the process.

The day we went in, I volunteered to go first, she was nervous, and I was ready. I drank a legal mind-altering concoction of lions-mane, cacao, cinnamon, black pepper, and turmeric, did some minor breathwork, sauna and cold plunge after my work out that A.M. and had completely surrendered to the woman performing the emotional code work. I was in the most open headspace I could have been at that time.

The first few readings were as I expected, suggestive, vague, and I imagine likely true for most people. But then she hit me with some shit that I couldn't handle. I'm standing there in front of this mysterious light worker, whom I had never met prior to this, Kaitlyn is in a seat beside me, I'm standing there, my eyes are closed, and the practitioner (Jamie) asks where there is a trapped emotion, what that trapped emotion is, and when I experienced it. You aren't supposed to answer verbally, you are just supposed to feel the answer as your energy communicates to her. When she asked when I experienced this emotion, I had a strong image come through, the emotion was intense abandonment. The image was a pair of white flat bottom sneakers, tight and light blue jeans shuffling down the sidewalk, I was staring straight down at them, feeling this massive rush of loneliness, abandonment, and overall disgusted feeling in myself and the people around me, for several seconds as Jamie continued to probe my energy for answers, I was just staring down feeling this way. These were not my shoes, these were women's jeans, legs, and sneakers.

She asked if this was an experience of my own, she got a quick no from the energies and then she asks if it is from the fathers' side, another quick no, she asks if it's from the mothers' side and I lost it. Completely, uncontrollably lost it. My eyes started sweating so bad it was almost embarrassing. In front of this stranger and my wife. In my minds' eye as she asks if it's a trapped emotion from the mothers' side, I simultaneously look up the street and then back over *my* shoulder, it's the town of Bellaire, where my mother grew up and where I lived a portion of my childhood. I recognize the bridge downtown, the buildings, they looked similar but different than the way I remembered them growing up. It was strange, I looked back down at my shoes shuffling and slightly stumbling over the sidewalk, looking back once more across the bridge and down toward my grandmother's home on the main street. I see her home in the distance and I feel a rush of energy like I've never felt in my life. I have never felt abandoned before, but in this moment, I felt completely abandoned.

She asks if it was from my mother, and then what age in which this occurred. She gets it narrowed down to somewhere between the ages of 17-19. At this time, I can hardly breath, I'm hyperventilating, and uncontrollably sweating from my eyeballs, like profusely, Kaitlyn is staring at me with this face like "Oh my God, what is going on? Is he okay? Am I going to be okay when it's my turn?"

My mother got pregnant with me at 18, I was born when she was 19. Her parents were previously divorced, and between the ages of 17 and 19 she had been kicked out of both her mothers' and her fathers' home. I couldn't put this into words at the time and still bringing up the scenario brings tears to my eyes. My mom never spoke of this time in her life. This was one of the most eye-opening sessions of my life.

We know that emotions are energy in motion and any energy that's motion is hindered or trapped can cause physical, mental, and spiritual damage. Like a bird to a window, abrupt stopping generally causes damage. Depending on the mass and velocity of the bird or emotion the more damage. We also know that our DNA holds on to a lot more information than just biological data. Fears, traumas, insecurities, passions, skills, and situational behavior can all be passed down. It serves as a survival mechanism, if Dad witnessed another member of the group get bitten and then die from a poisonous snake/spider he will likely hold on very tightly to that trauma and will avoid or kill those critters at all costs. This will be passed down to his offspring, as is the case with most of the human race. Dad learns fighting as a response to most of life's threats, his children receive this genetic response if it served the father in a beneficial way. Procreation in itself proves the benefit. Mom gets abandoned as a young woman, she copes with it, genetic information is stored and passed down, the offspring express independence as a positive result and detachment or unwillingness to pursue attachments as a negative result.

The emotional code healing process is supposed to heal the individual with the trapped emotion and whomever else holds trapped emotions due to this event. So naturally a few days after the session I asked my mom, who happened to be on her way to visit us with my grandfather (her father) at the time of the session, if she had noticed a feeling of any baggage coming off her shoulders. She was off put, of course, but intrigued. I asked if she had felt anything particularly refreshing on the day Kate and I did the session. She did. She said that while they were driving

213

to come visit, my father driving, her in the passenger seat and my grandfather in the back seat, he reached up and grabbed her shoulder, around the same time that I was being expelled of the awful emotion and said that he loved her. Held her shoulder for a second and that was it, she said that she had felt this strange sense of forgiveness and that her father never showed that type of adornment before. I told her about the vision and experience. She validated the shoes, the town as I saw it through her eyes, and her feelings. We both did that thing where our eyes get watery and stuff.

(Energy healing, Kaitlyn's emotional code experience)

Emotional Code is when you or an ancestor have not yet processed an emotion and it has been trapped in your energy field, which cause blockages or imbalances in your personal energy field. During this process you can permanently remove and release these emotions. The body is energy, we are made completely of energy from every atom that combines to create every cell, internal organ & bone. But it doesn't stop there, our thoughts, memories, consciousness, & emotions are all made of the same energy that makes the physical things we see and understand as *matter*. It is all made of pure energy. When you open your mind to viewing it from an energy standpoint you can see the effect of releasing trapped energy. Setting an emotion free from your energy field not only alleviates you but also any family member before or after you that this trapped emotion has affected is also free from its burden. It is wild I know!

This was my first time ever doing any type of spiritual work besides yoga, I was nervous, thankfully Trenton was already prepared to go first. At the time I was a little over 7 months pregnant with our 3rd beautiful baby and was interested in emotional code not just for me but for her as well. I had read that emotional code would release trapped emotions inside the body that were causing blockages and could manifest into larger blockages, deep debilitating fears and disease. I felt deeply drawn to do this for all three of our babes and myself as well. I watched Trenton & our healer set up shop, which was just standing in front of each other with complete relaxing, shoulders hang heavy, unclench the jaw, and attempt to bring peace to the body. As she entered in his energetic field, he was overcome with emotion many times, which he described previously. It was shocking to see him in these states, Trenton very rarely lets his emotions get the best of him like they had during this session, especially feelings of sadness. I have always prided him on being able to keep his composure so his lack of composure during this had me like "oh crap, this is going to be crazy!"

Before I knew it, it was my turn. I stood in front of the comfort & love of our healer and felt at ease but nervous at the same time. She started the journey into my energy field, I could feel emotions rising as she was picking up on different emotions and memories. I believe the first memory that was released was a memory from childhood that didn't have much effect on me, and I didn't even remember it happening. The second was around 12 and was a similar emotion this one I did feel and was a little bit uneasy, but it was cleared. The third trapped emotion was around mid-teenage years and this one I also felt but it was easy to let go of. My fourth trapped emotion was my early 20's this one was a little harsher because it was pretty recently trapped so I remembered feeling this way. Then out of nowhere it felt like my body was overtaken by a VERY strong emotion, I was completely terrified. I mean terrified to the point of crying so extremely hard that I started to dry heave, with a physical feeling of almost choking. I felt this deep, intense pit in my belly and an extreme clench in the abdomen... it just felt awful. I didn't totally receive images but intense emotions physically and mentally that had overtaken my body. I did however get a sense, I sensed that it was female but not my mother but close to me, she was younger in her 20's/early 30's & was in extreme fear of what I felt like was abuse of some sort.

Now after feeling this and the energy was cleared our healer had spoken with me and received info this emotion was ancestral, not one of mine but in fact came from my father's side, female. I was my beautiful grandmother's emotion that was trapped. This had me in awe that she had ever felt this way, also that it was carried TWO generations after to her granddaughter and maybe even her great granddaughters. With the release of this emotion from me, it is now released from everyone who would have carried it, so my father & our children.

I felt later this day sort of drained, the emotional toll it took on my body to experience such an intense emotion that had been hidden for a couple generations was harsh. Also feeling connected with my grandmother on a different level. Just so you can have a short visual on her, she was a beautiful "100%" little Italian lady with short almost black hair, tiny figure with deep brown eyes and at least one ring on every finger that she had always worn for as long as I can remember. Every Christmas she would put on the full show all by herself in the kitchen cooking up "Seven Fishes". My father, aunts & uncles would try to help her but she kind of didn't want them too, so she would always take over after they would attempt to help her. She was also the type of grandmother that HAND MADE all our easter candy every year, out of chocolate molds and created little bird nests out of candy for us. Although we did not see her much besides holidays and birthdays, she imprinted on me. She was the glue for the entire family on my father's side, keeper of all the drama & didn't share any of it, so I only knew my father's stories of being a child and what his childhood was like which was far different from mine.

I did not ask my dad that day if he felt any different because I thought he would've been so offput that I didn't think I would get the answer I was looking for, also I wanted to notice for my own eyes.

We stopped by later that day after the healing, talked with my dad on a few spiritual things that were right on topic that HE brought up. My dad will talk about anything & everything, but it was weird for him to bring it up pretty much right away. The sun was starting to set in late summer, so it was hot and humid but felt almost cooling. We started off talking about signs from spirits and how they come to visit us and let us know they are here. There was a light almost golden tone shining through my dad's eyes and he felt lighter to talk to in that moment. He mentioned his brother that had passed away the year prior & then mentioned my grandmother (his mom). He felt them while he was speaking of them, I could tell by his voice, honestly, I felt like I could feel them. I never told him that day what I had experienced but I could tell in his eyes and how he felt energetically that he felt her that day too. To me that was validating that it worked through him as well. *(Kaitlyn Sweet)*

Shamanic healing-soul retrieval was the next journey we went on outside of our own capabilities at the time. The ancient practice of soul retrieval brings back the beneficiary's soul or life force, pieces of which we lose throughout our life, specifically during traumatic or abusive events. Most of which tends to happen in our childhood since we have no understanding of how to handle these traumas or abuses yet, as we age, we build walls and create coping mechanisms that lessen the damage from similar instances. Parts of the soul leave the body and disassociate to protect itself from the pain. Not all traumas cause the soul to retreat, and some traumas that were seemingly miniscule compared to others were incidents where the soul fled to protect itself. Unconsciously a lot of your life force is spent searching for these soul parts so when they are returned you will feel whole and energized. If your life force is consistently depleted or is never returned you will find that you continue to attract similar traumatic incidents throughout your life. Resolving these traumas through the shamanic soul retrieval process will benefit you greatly.

Kate's shamanic healing story (Kaitlyn Sweet)

Trenton had gifted me with a shamanic healing "Soul Retrieval" service through the same healer that performed the emotional code healing. The goal of this process is to reconnect lost pieces of the soul that may have been lost prior in life. Welcoming them back home. I am sure we can all think of times in our life that we might had lost parts of ourselves in our life through traumatic events that had happened, but for me none of the events I could think of came up.

I had never done this type of healing before but was more knowledgeable and had done a lot more types of healing prior to this unlike my emotional code healing story. This was still a hard one for me to do! To be completely transparent when he bought it for me for Mother's Day I was upset! How could I be upset about receiving healing for myself? I felt so emotionally drained at this time because he was working super long hours & many MANY days in a row, and it seemed like it would never end. I felt like any type of additional work to my already full plate would probably crack my plate in half or just spill it all over the place (kind of dramatic but not). I immediately told him how I felt about it and looking back maybe I should have thought about it a few more times before I totally lost it on him and started to immediately go overboard, but hey that's how I felt at the time and how I needed to express myself. He was so shocked I felt this way and was supportive of me feeling this way but didn't quite get why I felt like it was adding to my chore list. Inner work can be hard, sometimes it takes me a few days to reset or even understand what the hell just happened and make sense of it or whatever other emotion comes up, but I am always SO THANKFUL I did it after words. It frees up space in my body and mind to take on new emotions and memories that are good for me and ultimately good for my family moving forward.

After a few days of thinking about what I wanted to do I decided to go for it and keep that appointment, I went in to meet my good friend who does the shamanic healing and is like an angel on earth. In the back of my mind, I was thinking worst case scenarios. What if something crazy comes up like there is darkness or something else crazy and unworldly like what the hell am I going to do with that? As I am in panic mode and having a super hard time putting my body in ease. It is kind of funny because before going into my experience I was thinking the literal absolute worst would happen, like deep demons would come out or things I buried and forgot that were so terrible I didn't remember because my body didn't want to... literally thinking the worst, and it was the exact opposite. I feared the word "Shamanic" and was a trained level 1 reiki healer, why?! I guess I had limiting beliefs on a word that someone somewhere had helped or taught me to believe. I grew up with strong affiliations with the church, my mother taught Sunday school and was a large part of the church when I was younger. A lot of my core values are that of the Christian faith, words like "shaman" still carried the "evil" like baggage with it that was wrongfully put there.

As I started my Shamanic journey I was smudged and laid down beside her connecting our feet and shoulders comfortably together with the sound of drum beating music in the background. I felt very comfortable and a little more at ease at least as much as I could let myself be, but I deeply trust her and know she would only do what was best for me.

Slowly but surely after about 20 minutes of drum music I finally could get to a place of not gulping and trying to hold my body still. Once I got here, I tried so hard to get meditative but couldn't help and wonder "where Is she" "who is she meeting" "is she seeing something crazy I did?" "Did she have to fight off a pack of crazy demons to get to my soul?" (It's so funny because I thought all this not yet knowing what Trenton would experience because I went first). It's a very vulnerable spot even with someone you deeply trust to open yourself up and be prepared for whatever they may uncover, but at the same time HOW AMAZING IS THAT. You can heal yourself with the help of someone else or even by yourself (if you've been trained and practice the skill.)

The drum music had stopped, she came out of her meditation and grabbed her journal (it's like a dream so she immediately needs to write the info before she loses it) she began to write the timeline and what she experienced and proceeded to say, "That was wild I have not experienced something like that before."

She told me that my future self-met her in my shamanic healing to help guide her through my healing processes and what needed healing!! What the heck, wait so future me, met past me… and healed through present me?! She responded "Yeah you walked me through and even spoke with me on the subject, you were confident, older, polished and successful." I was quite literally blown away by hearing this, especially with my prior roller coaster to making it to this point. My future self-helped guide her to the point in my past (but present) life that needed to be fixed emotionally. A few situations were young, like less than 8, some in later teenage years, but one stuck out the most in the soul retrieval, I was about middle school age when I had a deep story, she was able to describe it vividly, a teacher purposefully picking on me in front of the classroom and deeply embarrassed me and made me feel small and insignificant. She said this teacher was sick mentally and had his own problems outside of work, but I didn't understand that at the time and I let this man value my self-worth. Being so young at that weird age in middle school, it hit me deeply so much, so that a part of my soul quite literally left that day. It was a big part of my soul as well and something I delt with in the back of my head DAILY, something that I had fought against with little gain ever since that moment.

We were able to re- write the story for myself, with the help of my beautiful future self, there to talk to the healer and my beautiful younger self through it. Isn't this experience completely out of this world!? As I'm typing this experience out, I still can't completely wrap my head around the whole story. I do know time is irrelevant in the quantum field… But until you experience something so "not normal" to your everyday life, you don't really get it, at least I didn't. I am at what I feel like is just the tip of the iceberg with healing, when I thought I had already mastered it. Healing & health goes so deeply and has so many avenues. It's not just food, diet, exercise, sunlight, grounding, laughing, emotion, memories, thoughts, routines, past lives... etc. It's quite literally EVERYTHING and everything is energy. I am on the journey of self-healing and finding my deeper connection to serving every day and the shamanic soul retrieval process has lit up a world I once perceived as darkness, I can't wait to see what else I can learn about energy. *(Kaitlyn Sweet)*

After Kate did her journey into shamanic healing, she set me up to do the same. I was nervous but a lot less speculative since the last experience was so vivid. I was more worried about what type of memories and situations from my past the shaman (Jamie) was going to witness. I was afraid to be embarrassed more than anything else. I drank my special *"it's okay, I'm open and receptive to this modality"* nootropic concoction and went in with as little fear as I could. The ceremony starts with a short description as the shaman feels out my mood, she gives me a quick energy pat down (burning sage around me to cleanse my aura) prior to beginning. She starts the drums and begins putting herself in a trance while we lay down together and touch elbows and ankles side by side (so that she can connect more rapidly and easily to my soul/energy). I relax as much as I can, just praying to my higher self that certain parts of my past that may have been traumatic and embarrassing, stay between me and my spirit guides, promising that I would handle them later, on my own. Thirty minutes or so go by, the drumming stops, she sits up and begins writing in her journal, shamans describe their experience as dream-like, so they write down their experience quickly afterwards so that, like a dream, they don't forget too quickly.

I went to the restroom for a moment afterwards and took my time returning hoping that her experience retrieving parts of my soul was like Kate's where she met with Kate's future self and she was banging hot, rich, and spiritually inclined enough to walk the shaman through the healing process. As it turns out, at least for this first experience, there was deeper work to be done. She informed me that I had been battling a dark energy my entire life. An energy that she described as a large, dark, storm cloud that she had to clear out of the way for most of the session before she could attempt to retrieve parts of my soul. I was always told that everyone dealt with the same kind of demons and temptations as I had, but apparently the extent of this isn't the same for all of us. I had conditioned myself to believe that I just needed to be more mentally tough to handle the dark side. Which in part, is the reason for many of the mindful fitness strategies that I developed and incorporate in my daily life. I was a bit shocked but also relieved to know that the energy had been released. It explained a lot for me, the abuse I inflicted on my own mind, body and soul was powerful, the coping mechanisms had led to addictions, some actions and some substances, and those addictions, although I defeated long before this were always looming around me, tempting me at every corner. Since this ceremony, those temptations have disappeared.

I know that this might sound crazy and that's because it is. At least through the lenses of our current culture. A culture that has been built around the denial of miracles, health, wealth, and strength coming from within a person, a culture that teaches people that they are *without* these traits and abilities and that they need to acquire them from an outside source. Our culture

223

may have evolved into a business, but we still possess much of our primal knowledge. Unlock, and awaken this knowledge within you and believe in the power of spiritual energy, utilize awakened souls around you in your own awakening.

Everyone is a shaman

I am a believer in energy, soul, and spirit. I believe that at our cores each human being has the power to heal themselves and others. Some people are more open, able to let that energy flow through their physical bodies without obstructing it or their own capacity to channel it. I believe that we are all born with psychic, healing, and intuitive abilities but as we grow, these traits are lost. Not because they are not important skills to keep but because our modern culture downplays and discredits these abilities. Calling them "witchcraft", "magic", "fairy tales", "Make-believe", or just plain rubbish. Parents often tell their kids that they aren't seeing or hearing anything when they stare off at something or ask about something that no one else can see, they tell them that they are wrong and that they can't do things, children are told that healing comes from a special person and their pills and procedures that they offer rather than from within. When they see colors surrounding people (auras), speak of people we have never heard of, or situations that we know weren't from this lifetime, when they talk about places that they have never been, most parents just tell them they are wrong and don't ask them to elaborate or explore those memories. Our kids have said some astonishing things to my wife and I that they could never know unless they were connected spiritually. Why can't it be believed that they are? Quantum entanglement literally describes how every atom in the entire universe from the moment of the big bang, is entangled (intertwined) with every other atom in the universe. That means that everything, is attached to everything at the most basic level. Not only is everything made up of energy, but all that energy is connected. No matter the distance.

My best friend died last September and after he died my son would sometimes stare off at something normally above and beside my head and ask me "Is Harvey your Friend? Is he dead?" and I would say "Yeah buddy, he passed away." He would keep staring and ask me "Where do people go when they pass away?" normally he would follow that question with something like "Is he here? Or in heaven?". He would keep his stare always, intently above and beside my head like he was looking at something. I never knew exactly how to answer his questions so I would tell him that "yes he passed away, and your body dies, I believe that your soul is able to travel wherever it wishes, so Harvey might be in heaven, or here, or with his kids, it's really hard to say unless you can see or feel him? I always tried to dig a bit deeper into what Wade was feeling but he would normally just continue with his four-year-old life and toys.

When Harvey passed away, I was in the middle of really digging deep into my mind about past sufferings and experiences that were weighing me down. When he died the soul searching got deeper and my children's' clairvoyance made it especially difficult. A lot of times I would get random thoughts and feelings, sometimes goosebumps out of no-where and thoughts of other passed loved ones or memories would flood my mind, then one of the kiddos or both would reassure the feeling. Making me feel connected and blessed. Our son Wade and oldest daughter Maelyn both believe without a doubt that they know great grandparents that died long before they were born. Even before I was born. Maelyn once said that she chose Kate to be her mommy. That she chose me to be her daddy before she was in mommy's belly. This sort of thing could be born from an active imagination, but where does a child get the idea of choosing their family, or being anywhere before being where they are now?

I don't know exactly how all this works, but Kate and I can both attest to this, when we are at our most open, vulnerable, and accepting states of mind for spiritual enlightenment, our kids are too. It's like our energy amplifies their natural abilities.

If you have children, do them and yourself a favor. Listen to them, observe them, be WITH them. Don't discredit any of their wild questions, statements, or ideas. They might just be on to something heavenly. Sometimes it might be entirely bull crap but who cares. Entertain it with your entire mind.

"Put down what you are carrying"
Trevor Hall

If I didn't just "Woo Woo" you right out of this book, then we can explore the question of why energy clearing and stabilizing is important. Ancient people believed that there existed multiple energy centers within the human body. You can call them energy centers or chakras if you prefer. They exist in the most energy dense areas of our physical bodies. It is believed that if these energies are not working in coherence with the other energies and are not flowing smoothly, the function of the physical body will suffer. The soul and mind will also suffer. The major energy centers are just above your head, slightly above and between your eyes, the middle of your throat, the center of your chest, your solar plexus between your heart and navel, your sacrum, and your root at the perineum.

Emotions in the modern world are not always expressed exactly as they are felt internally, many primal or deeply rooted human emotions are suppressed. Like the urge to laugh hysterically in a meeting when someone says something ridiculous, to be-little your boss when their head gets too big, to show your true compassion and passion, to show your true love to someone, to show aggression when you are frustrated, or to show vulnerability of any kind. This is what a trapped emotion is. You feel an overwhelming amount of stress because of modern life, you fear so many things, but you can't express any of them. Because you are supporting a family, you must stay strong and resilient. I've been there, these energies must go into motion at some point, or they will create blockages in the flow of your life energy. Don't let any trapped emotions stop you from being a tranquil warrior, supporting your spouse as a tranquil warrior or from raising tranquil warriors.

Trapped energies will keep you from being the best of version of yourself. You can be a health nut in every other aspect of your life and still develop cancer, simply because your energy is off. You can do everything else in this book and still not be the version of you that God intended if you aren't expressing and releasing all your emotions. I *love* to let out a primal yell sometimes when I'm alone, a yell of excitement, anger, mourning, hell it doesn't matter, just a yell. A loud and proud roar, from my gut. Like a fucking wolf or tiger. It feels good. Try it. Before you judge the practice, give it a try. Next time you are alone and feel comfortable, just let it out. You *will* feel a rush of emotions, you will feel ignited. I keep this as a part of my

227

weekly practice just in case for some reason I didn't let out some excitement.

There are energy workers all over the world that can help guide you to the water, but they cannot make you drink. That, you must do on your own. If you don't have an open mind on the topic then don't waste your time because it will not work. Awakening is a journey, for most people it takes years, decades, or even a lifetime to complete. Some people never fall asleep. Some people awaken accidentally. I am uncovering my tranquil warrior little by little.

My practice beyond the integral primal yell includes a mix of breathwork, meditation, intense exercise, sauna sessions, and ice plunging. Not necessarily in that order. Personally, defeating the body first allows me to open my mind and spirit much more easily. When all else fails, or when you just need further help, reiki, kundalini yoga, emotional code, shamanic practices, past life trauma healing, therapy, energy clearing, sound baths, ancestral medicinal drugs, etc. are always there as well. Find what fits best with the time you have, find what practices are the easiest for you to stick with and what practices are enjoyable to you. Just remember that it is all on you, nobody else can "save" you from you, that's your responsibility.

CHAPTER SEVEN

AWAKENING A LIMITLESS LIFE, YOU VS. YOU

Maybe you weren't lucky enough to have someone in your childhood tell you that you could be anything you ever wanted to be. Or maybe you are like almost every other child and even though someone did tell you that, you didn't believe it. Or something shut you down later in life when you attempted to be what you wanted to be. Whatever the case, I bet that of the 70,000 or so thoughts you have every day, most of them are telling yourself what you can't or shouldn't do, what you didn't or won't do. Things that you can't or won't have. Or you reflect those feelings outwardly towards other people you see, jealousy and spitefulness are just other ways of telling yourself that you aren't good enough. When was the last time you told yourself good job? I'm proud of myself, I am… insert compliment. Most of us are our own worst enemies when it comes to limiting self-talk. These limiting beliefs hold us back from achieving all the things that we truly desire. We are worth it; YOU are worth it.

Think about how lucky you are to be here today. Of the millions of sperm cells that could have made it to one of the 40 thousand or so eggs, you made it. Creating just one cell. Surviving as that single cell and growing into 40 trillion cells. From that first cell to birth was a long journey for you, you were lucky to be conceived but even luckier to be born. You were lucky enough to be born somewhere where someone loved you enough to keep you alive long enough for you to learn how to read. You are lucky to have grown up to whatever age you may currently be. You are lucky each morning you wake up. You are lucky to live in a country where you are free to read whatever you want. You are lucky to take each breath. You are lucky that your soul chose your body, that your spirit guides choose to stay with you. YOU ARE LUCKY.

You are unique, you are special. Your personality is yours and yours alone. There are no matching fingerprints or brains in this universe past or present. Your experiences are yours. Your thoughts are yours. You are unique and special. Just being you is a contribution to the world. You are enough. Okay, okay, So if you're so damn special, then why don't you act like it?

A teacher, coach, peers, or a parent's opinion can change the way we feel about ourselves. I bet you can recall at least one moment where one of those influencers above said something negative to or about you that gave you a limiting self-belief. Think about that moment for a bit. Wouldn't it feel good to let that moment go?

Let's do a quick exercise, recall that moment again and work through the following questions. Why would they say or do that? Were they in a rough patch in their life? Jealous, vindictive? Did they mean to hurt you as much as they did? Maybe they were suffering through their own demons and took it out on you, maybe they didn't even mean what they said. Find a reason why. Now think of how sorry you are for them; it really must've been hard for them dealing with all those demons. Think about how that moment led you here, to this book. How it led to you changing your life for the better. Without their comment or action, you wouldn't be here today. Thank them for that.

Chances are, they don't remember the moment, and if they do, they probably didn't mean to cause legitimate trauma. The way that we treat other people reflects how we treat ourselves.

Now that you've gone through this realization you can move forward. If you are like me, you can find MANY circumstances where someone tried and succeeded in bringing you down. And I have always been very headstrong, believing 100% that no one could ever hurt me. I felt like my pride and mind were impenetrable like a heavily guarded castle with a giant mote full of alligators surrounding it. Sticks and stones baby, words had no effect on me. And I never showed that they did either. As a new chapter of my life was unfolding, I realized that my indestructible ego had taken some heavy hits along the way. Once I started exploring my memories, I found that I had a lot of work to do. If you find yourself dwelling on those memories, it's time to process them. Find the positivity in them, realize that they are just people too. Maybe we are that person to someone else. Something we said or did that created a limiting belief in someone else. If you can recall being that person, apologize for dumping your emotions on to them and inflicting emotional pain. Then, forgive yourself. Give yourself time to work through these thoughts, don't overwhelm yourself by taking on your entire history at once.

The other part of limiting self-beliefs is that the brain wants nothing more than to be fed, in control and to live. This brain sees a LOT of dangers out there in the world. One of those dangers is your ability to act out of a consciousness that might go against that happy place of homeostasis. In ancestral times this mechanism probably served us well more regularly, in the modern world there are too many dangerously convenient ways to stay out of what our brain understands as dangers way. It recognizes things that make us uncomfortable as dangerous and wants to avoid those things at all costs. Our brain is such a powerful organ that as we starve to death, our brain will literally break down the nutrients and calories from other organs like our own heart before letting itself starve. Cruel, and often what it is perceiving as dangerous isn't even remotely life threatening. It reassures us constantly through those 70,000 or so thoughts per day that we are inadequate and should not proceed with new experiences or with experiences that harmed its ego in the past.

During the writing of this book, I have been engaged in constant battle with my ego and my protective brain. My soul was awakening this tranquil warrior, I was beginning to understand much more about myself and the world around me. I was becoming more capable of handling stress and was understanding that the path I was on, was not the path that I wanted to travel. It had led me here, but the direction that path was headed, was not the destination in which I wanted to arrive. At the onset of writing this book, 100-hour work weeks were the norm. I was waking up at 1:30 AM and driving 2 hours each way to work my 12-hour shift (a 12-hour shift in a position that I had worked very hard to get to and have been doing for six years, 12 years total in various positions), I never knew when I would have time off, sometimes I was needed to work extra hours, sometimes even double shifts or triple shifts, I would be called out sometimes just hours after I had left. For the effort though, the money was great, really great. I was the man on the work site, when I showed up to start a job people literally flocked around my truck to talk to me and help me with whatever I needed. I was the guy to solve any issues, I was *the guy*. My ego got fluffed every single day. The job was difficult, I had to constantly prove my worth and intelligence to the customers I worked for, but I loved the look on an old dude's face with 40 years of experience when I could solve a problem quickly and easily. For a long time, the money and the ego fluffing were enough to keep me working hard day in and day out, the sacrifices seemed worth it. To my comfortable and survival-oriented brain, it was worth it.

In the background though, my life was falling apart. My life's greatest blessings were beginning to fade away and somehow, I was stuck in this limbo of "my job provides, I need this job, we need this job, without this job blah blah blah" and "I need out, I hate this job, we can't live like this, this job is ruining my life". I believed unequivocally that I couldn't leave my job, but I simultaneously *had* to leave my job. The stress was all but tearing me apart, and during this limbo I ruptured my plantar fascia in my left foot (the foot related to being or feeling stuck). I had a true passion for health and fitness my whole life and in my career in the oil and gas industry, I wrote many nutrition plans and workout regimens for co-workers (and still have several of them as clients today). I talked for countless hours with people about health and wellness, I would often have groups of people at my tailgate eating raw liver, bone marrow, and fruits they had never heard of before. While talking about the benefits of each. I started many pushup and pullup competitions on site, I would have people try to perform heavy lifts with the kettlebells that I had brought from home or trying to pick up heavy items around the work site. People watched me workout shirtless in the middle of the day on work site and occasionally join in. Fitness is something I truly love and has always been a huge part of me. I always had this urge to awaken people to how bad ass they could really be. But I never saw it as a full-time career, I didn't believe that I could make as much money in the fitness industry as I did where I was.

As our children started to get older it became abundantly clear to me that my love for Kaitlyn and our kids was far greater than the love for my work. When it was just Kate and I things were simpler, the long days and hours were easier to recuperate from, and we could travel together for work and as difficult as it was, it was still manageable. We could still spend enough time together and focus on one another, we could love deeply and enjoy time off together. When you have children, you need to give them everything, all your attention, love, support, and guidance. But you also need to give all of this to your spouse. And somewhere in the mix you need to give those things to yourself. When you are raising three young children and working 100 + hours a week this is difficult. It's not like Kaitlyn didn't have stuff going on either and was this 1950s housewife that just took care of the kids and house. She owns and operates an online clothing store, had a wedding hair business, helped me with the nutrition programs for co-workers and online clients, was going to yoga and reiki school, reading daily, was raising the kids, taking care of the household chores, and was still working out on a regular basis.

We were making the best of the situation; I would get home around 6:00 and she would rush to a fitness class. I would play with the kids for a bit while doing dishes, cooking dinner and meal prepping for myself for the next workday. When Kaitlyn got home, we would eat dinner as a family. Then I would work out quickly in the garage gym and finish with an ice plunge and/or sauna session while Kate cleaned up from dinner and got the kids ready for bed. When I finished, I would read or tell the kids stories, tuck them in bed and then I would prepare my coffee, clothes, salt-water etc. for the morning, shower if I felt the need and then Kaitlyn and I would talk for a few minutes as we fell asleep. Just to wake up at 1:30 AM and do it all again. Sometimes for several weeks at a time. In the mean-time home repairs needed done, the grass still needed cut, grocery shopping needed done, the ducks needed taken care of and a plethora of other daily duties to squeeze in.

As the kids grew, I noticed a few things. One, Kaitlyn was forced to put a lot of her dreams and aspirations on a shelf, she felt as though she couldn't pursue her goals as fully as she wanted to. Two, my children were acting out towards her when I was working, because they needed more attention. Their wants, needs, and dreams were also being put up on a shelf. Three, my dreams were on a shelf. And the final thing I realized was that all this struggle was getting us nowhere. In fact, we were falling apart. Things had to change, but just the thought of change had my brain in panic mode "how will we pay the bills? How will we buy groceries? How will we etc. etc. etc." We so desperately needed a life change, but my brain so desperately wanted to keep doing the same thing. Even though it wasn't working. My job made me feel safe and secure in a lot of ways. But was also starting to tear apart the things that I wanted to keep safe and secure. Overcoming this fear was the hardest thing I have ever done.

Looking back at all the parties, holidays, events, funerals, and other extremely important activities in our lives that I missed because of my recent career I realize that it has made every event I have been able to attend, and each one I will attend moving forward even more important. When you miss out on things, it makes you appreciate them more. I *knew* I was doing the right thing by choosing to provide instead of attend, but I was making the wrong choice. I wasn't needed away from my family; I was needed where my family was.

We took a leap of faith. We had to. If we wanted to stay together as a strong family, if we wanted to continue being a happy family, we had to dive in headfirst to a new chapter. Ultimately, I had to let go of the false sense of security that my job provided, and Kate had to let go of the independence and resentment she had built up over the years. Kate and I always worked as a great team, but we worked as a great team from two very different locations. We share many of the same passions and wanted to work together but we weren't sure how. So, we decided to collaborate on this book, collaborate in teaching fitness classes, and are opening a gym together. Energy Fitness Studio in the south hills of Pittsburgh. The new chapter of our life has been coming together the way we wanted it to, and we have been happier ever since taking the leap. The hardest decision I have ever made in my life has become the best decision I have every made in my life.

Breaking habits and changing the law

Do you know the law of attraction? What you perceive is what you believe and what you believe is what you conceive. Meaning that your perceptions create your reality. If nine out of ten of your daily thoughts or 63,000 thoughts a day are preventing you from progressing, then you probably won't be progressing any time soon. Correcting just half of your daily thoughts are going to improve the quality of your work and life by more than you can imagine. The harder you work at regaining control of your thoughts the faster you will regain control of your mind and thus changing your past, present and future tremendously.

Yes, I said past. Because as you begin to perceive and believe your past experiences from new perspectives you conceive a new memory of those events. A new understanding will inevitably lead to a new future.

How do you do it? Next time you catch yourself in the middle of one of these limiting thoughts, laugh at yourself. "Almost got me again, ha-ha" sounds silly but the more often you call your brain on its bullshit the less it will affect you, and the less often those thoughts will appear. If you feel like you need extra clarification after you call out the bullshit, give yourself an example of why it isn't true any ways. Here is an example from my personal experience. My limiting brain- "You can't write a book, you have way too much going on." My awakened consciousness- "Wow, fuck you brain. I hope you know that we are in this together, you better help me write this book." True story, maybe not word for word but you get the picture. And that's my brain after years of training it. I am aware that my brain doesn't intend on hurting me with these limiting thoughts, it is only doing its job. Every time before I jump into my ice tub at home or a freezing cold body of water there is a similar conversation that happens, "I don't need to plunge today I did it the other day, it's gonna be so cold!" as I overcome the fear peddler inside my own head and dunk myself in freezing cold water, submerge my head and hold my breath as long as I can, surface and then capture my breath, and smile. Each time I do this I defeat that voice and regain control. Just remember that as crazy as it may sound, we all have these thoughts, we all question our own abilities, even though we have won so many battles in the past.

Here are a few tricks that have helped me with mental toughness and stability. Start by doing things that make you uncomfortable on purpose. Face your fears head on. What's something that practically everyone feels uncomfortable with? The cold. Especially extreme cold. So, my favorite mental toughness trick is the ice plunge. You can do this in a handful of ways, find a cold body of natural water and jump in it. Submerge your head for 20-30 seconds and then *chill* in the water with as much of your body as you can under the water for a few minutes. If its summertime or you don't have access to a local body of water, then turn the water in your shower all the way to cold and duck your head under for 20-30 seconds and again, just chill for a few minutes. There are a few companies that sell specific tubs for this purpose. Or you can buy a trough, barrel, or vessel that you can comfortably fit in. (I bought a 100-gallon plastic trough from tractor supply.) Fill it up with water (your hose water should be roughly 55*) and add 66lbs or so of ice (depending on the ambient temperature, you are aiming for 40* or less water temp), jump in, with your head submerged for 20-30 seconds and chill for a few minutes. 55* degree water is cold, so for beginners I recommend getting comfortable with the temperature of the water coming out of the tap before adding ice to your regimen. After the full body submersion soak for a bit, I prefer the range between 3-5 minutes. This works to break down that control your brain has over keeping you from doing new and potentially uncomfortable things. Your brain is going to say "No!" every time you go to plunge yourself into the ice. But every time you respond to your brain with a powerful "Yes!" and jump in, you are taking control. There are countless reasons to enjoy ice plunges on a regular basis but for the simple purpose of reducing limiting beliefs it's my go to. I often wonder, if I hadn't been training my mind for years to overcome uncomfortable situations, would I have been able to quit my career and pursue my dreams?

The benefits of ice plunging are . . .

- Increased mental, physical, and emotional resilience
- Increased health span
- Increased testosterone and libido
- Increased recovery time for hard bouts of exercise
- Increased metabolism
- Increased energy levels
- Protects against muscle atrophy
- Boosts mood
- Boosts immune system
- Stress management
- Improves the quality of your sleep
- Helps stave off cognitive decline

Another intensely stressful mental toughness trick is heat therapy. You can achieve this by exercising in the hot sun during summer, or you can use a sauna. Sauna use can work just as well as a high intensity cardio session, minus the damage to joints and time because it elevates your heart rate and maintains that higher rate while releasing muscle protecting proteins, so you are getting recovery and exercise in one. Using this in contrast to your cold therapy is phenomenal to your health and mental stability. Find a place that has saunas, build, or buy your own sauna. Get it fired up to 140 degrees or better and get uncomfortable. Just 57 minutes per week has been shown to provide health benefits (Soeberg et al, 2021). Heat and cold therapies offer many of the same benefits as the other. For mental toughness results it doesn't really matter if it's a dry sauna, infrared sauna or whatever it just matters that its hot. Drink lots of mineral enriched water, add Himalayan or Celtic Sea salt to your water, eat hydrating foods before and after sauna use. Be careful to not overdue the heat initially as most people will need to build a tolerance but at the same time don't wuss out on yourself. Know your TRUE limits, not those ones that your fear mongering brain is setting.

We purchased our sauna from "The Sauna Guys" out of the Upper Peninsula of Michigan. This sauna has held rock steady since day one, and we use it (as a family and just my wife and I) at least four times a week. I highly recommend wooden built, barrel, wood stove saunas like the ones they hand make but you can also find indoor saunas that are electric. Electric saunas heat up a lot faster and you can get them in different infra-red-light frequencies, blue tooth speakers and the whole deal. We prefer the old school wood stove smell and feel to the modern saunas though. I also enjoy cutting wood, to me it counts as extra activity, helps me connect to nature and feels more natural.

Lastly, exercise. Specifically, for me is the early morning exercise. Waking up before the sun rises, long before anyone else wakes up. Just getting yourself out of bed at 4 or 5am is a struggle, especially on days off. Defeating the "sand man" adds to your mental toughness. Your brain will obviously try to keep you in bed if possible. You are in control, you want to get stronger and more fit, you want to be a better version of yourself. When your inner voice starts saying things like "five more minutes" or "I worked out yesterday", it's time to get up. Don't let your brain get in your way. It doesn't matter the modality in which you like to train, just make sure that you are moving your body in ways that contradict your regular day to day life and that you keep it varied.

The key to overcoming your primal brain truly is just facing those fears. Public speaking? Exposing your sensitivity? Admitting you're wrong? Complimenting someone else? When you feel yourself backing out of something think "Is there a good reason or is my brain just acting out of instinct again?". Often that will be the case.

CHAPTER EIGHT

ACTIVATING YOUR TRANQUIL WARRIOR
THROUGH MOVEMENT

I saved this chapter for last because this is what ties the reparation of human health and the development of warrior like tranquility all together. We are a multi-faceted being, meaning that we function on many different levels. A temporary level being our vessel or temple and an energetic and infinite level. Our body and our soul. But life as a human being as we have discussed is a bit more complicated, our soul has motives, passions, abilities, wants and needs and is temporarily attached to our body. While our body has many different functions, passions, abilities, motives, wants and needs as well. Then of course there's the wants and needs of our ego and shadow sides. Oftentimes these wants and needs are not unified. Reconnecting to nature, food, environmental stressors, ancestral & spiritual practices, realigning your energy centers and developing a mindful fitness routine will get you well on your way. The last, and most important thing you can do for the health of your temple is move it.

Active lifestyles have become a thing of the past. Just a few generations ago most of the work was done manually and outdoors in the sunshine. People also got to work in a more laborious way. Walking, riding a horse or bicycle, etc. Modern people sit on their way to work in a comfortable vehicle, spend countless hours per day sitting at work, then sit on the way home from work, sit down to eat dinner and/or watch tv, then go lay down in bed. That is not what I would call an active lifestyle. Working out at your local gym for an hour three times a week obviously increases your activity level but only 3 more hours out of the 168 available. The hours spent training in the gym are not wasted, but if you want to maximize the quality of your life you are going to have to increase your overall activity level. "Pain avoidance is a powerful motivator for mediocrity. "*Living Fully Pod Cast.*

That means that your life needs to be active. Our early ancestors remained healthy and fully functional into their late 50's and 60's despite never taking a pill, getting a hip replacement or a set of dentures. No question that every other topic covered in this book relates to that resilience, but the consistent movement is also a necessary part of the equation. Humans seem to be designed to live around 80 years before cellular senescence kicks into overdrive, something that Scientists like the Author of "Lifespan" David A Sinclair are working on mitigating through breakthrough medical science. Daily low intensity movements kept our ancestors active all the time outside of high intensity hunting and no intensity sleeping. Activities like walking rougher terrain than your city sidewalk, squatting down, lunging, twisting, climbing trees, throwing things, kept them young and robust throughout their lives.

Our early ancestors on the African grasslands began as scavengers and foragers, then became persistent hunters and gathers. Eventually becoming less persistent and more efficient. This is one of the reasons they shed the body hair for sweat glands. Humans are quite small compared to our first and longest lasting food source, the bovine. Male aurochs (the ancestor of modern cows') were roughly 10.2 feet long, 6 feet tall, and over

3,300 lbs. with a set of 2 ½ feet long and 8-inch-thick horns. In comparison a modern bull is about 8 feet 2 inches long, 5 feet 5 inches tall, and weighing about 2,000 lbs. A couple pokes with a spear or arrows would not have killed the ancient beast where it stood. Groups of hunters would need to injure the animal and then follow it as it fled until if finally collapsed and then they could harvest the beast. Once killed, the harvest would need to be packed back to the rest of the tribe adding a heavy load hike to the end of their marathon that was preceded by a high intensity fight. These groups of hunters could be compared to painted wolves or African dogs as they follow an injured prey for many hours until they can finally bring it down easily. Human beings are designed to endure long periods of moderate intensity a few times a week with positive results. We did so for roughly 2 million years. This appears to be a use it or lose it scenario as is most everything fitness related. If you enjoy jogging or running, try adding some slower paced jog intervals and fast paced sprinting and running in the mix to really use what biology has given you. The same can be done swinging a kettlebell, swimming or on a rowing machine, bicycle, heavy bag etc.

When it comes to sprinting, high intensity plyometric exercise should not be the bulk of your regimen unless you are training to beat Usain Bolts records. But you should incorporate some maximum effort movements into your life. Jumping should not be the bulk, nor should yoga, long distance running, or heavy resistance training unless of course you are training for the sake of career or monetary gain. If you are "training" to enjoy a longer, healthier, and happier life it is important to have a goal or focus but it is equally important to break up the monotony and move your body in *all directions* with all applied forces. This

245

will keep you motivated, rested, healed, and ready for the next challenge. Love yoga, jogging, clanging plates in the gym, swinging kettlebells, boxing, sprinting, jumping on boxes? Great! But the human body is not designed to lift massive amounts of weight or endure massive amounts of high intensity impacts on a daily basis. Nor is it designed to sit around all day. The human body *is* designed to adapt and overcome obstacles though, so yes lifting heavy three or more times a week will build strength, doing yoga three times a week will increase core strength and flexibility, jogging three times a week will increase cardiovascular function, etc. etc. But there are ways to accomplish certain goals without destroying your body and spending multiple hours every day in the gym. Hit the sauna a few times a week to simulate a cardio session, ice plunges to increase cardiovascular function without even pounding a single mile of pavement. Park your car further away from the entrance of the store, cook with cast iron pans & skillets (not only for the health benefit of discarding nonstick but also the weight of the pan! (Kaitlyn)) there are so many things you can do in your daily life that make it slightly less convenient but so much better for your body.

We are also designed to conserve energy. If you move at a slow pace for most of the day with a few hours of moderate intensity and short bouts here and there of high intensity your body will adapt, and your physical fitness will improve. Hit the gym as often as you like, or even more, just make sure that you are adequately nourishing and recovering from hard bouts of exercise. If you really want to be the best version of yourself then you need to move more often throughout the day and treat yourself to some short bouts of exercise periodically. Sneak away from your work area every hour or so and do some pushups, air squats, pullups, planks etc. Walk around during your lunch break and if you can, get outside in the fresh air and sunshine.

You think I'm being unrealistic? I used to bring kettlebells and bands with me to work, every few hours or so (when I could sneak away) I would stand behind my pick-up and put in 5-10 minutes' worth of swinging, snatching, cleaning etc. I would find something to do pullups on and a clean spot to do pushups. Often people would see me doing this and it would lead to mini competitions and many a nay-sayer jumped on the "get healthier" band wagon. Don't be ashamed, the people that will pick fun at you for bettering yourself aren't on your side anyways. Some will disapprove and others will join you. Each day should include an actual planned gym/studio etc. session. An hour(ish) dedicated to exercise, a large part of the day walking and moving, and what Ben Greenfield calls "exercise snacks" sprinkled in throughout the day.

An exercise snack is a quick bout of high to moderate intensity exercise that gets your heart rate up and a decent burn/muscle pump. A set of a body weight exercises 60%-75% of your maximum limit will do the trick. If you can perform 10 pullups then do 6-7 of them, if you can perform 25 pushups then do 15-18. Pushups, planks, pullups, air squats, lunges, burpees etc. I am a huge fan of exercising and always have been, even when I was fat, I was still *strong*. This might come as a surprise to most people but moving your body is fun. It is natural, and no, it shouldn't hurt. If it does hurt, that is a signal. A signal that something needs attention. Use it or lose it, move what hurts. Move it a little bit every day, every few hours, every hour, all the time until it stops hurting and you then can start adding resistance. If you tell your body that your *bum* knee is useless, that's what it is. If you tell your body that you need that knee and it isn't useless, that's what it is. Your body will adapt, utilize all the other information in this book and include daily movement, you will improve your life on many planes. Some injuries require more attention than that. But for your daily aches and pains, move the heck out of them.

Exercise has always been an integral part of my life. I enjoy moving my body both meditatively and with high intensity. Through the years I have learned a great deal about my own body and what types of training work best for me. I have learned a great deal more through personal training, everyone reading this book has a different background, different set of goals, different styles of training that they enjoy and different body types that react different to each modality. What works best for me in the gym doesn't always work best for the next person. I recommend creating a specific set of personal goals and make those goals your main objective in the gym. Diversify your program and make it fun, incorporate group classes or sports/activities so that you will stay accountable. Join some competitions, events, or teams if you have the time. Hiking, biking, swimming, basketball, tennis, volleyball, yoga, tai chi, whatever just have fun with your life. If your specific goal is to get huge or ripped, then you will have to specify your gym routine. Incorporate everything you have learned in this book and make living healthy fun. If you need a personal trainer and holistic nutritionist that are equipped to awaken your inner tranquil warrior don't hesitate to reach out to myself or Kaitlyn. You can find us on Instagram @The_Tranquil_Warrior and @Katies_Sweet or you can reach out to us at EnergyFitnessStudios.com

If you enjoyed this book, please give us a share and a tag on social media!

Key Points

o Processed sugar is an addictive substance, treat it as such.
o Expose lots of your bare skin to the sun every day.
o Unplug as often as possible.
o Get grounded in nature daily.
o Stop disinfecting everything all the damn time.
o Stop engaging in emotional addictions.
o Release and recover from trapped emotions.
o Trust your community, be a part of a community.
o Engage in a boundless mentality.
o Let go of limiting belief systems.
o Don't give in to short term dopamine kicks while forgoing your future goals. The future will inevitably show up.
o Get comfortable being uncomfortable.
o Move your body like your ancestors.
o Lunge, twist, hinge, squat, jump, climb, MOVE.
o Engage your brain in new and creative ways.
o What you consume determines who you are. This includes news, tv, radio, social media, food, skin care products, toilet paper, pets, energy, emfs, people around you...

TRANQUIL WARRIOR TASKS

- Eliminate processed sugar
- Eliminate seed oils
- 30 minutes of direct sunlight with at least 50% bare skin
  - 50% is debatable but to me it means, face, neck, shoulders down to your hands, knees down and feet. Get comfortable with less clothes on. Your confidence is VERY IMPORTANT.
- 30 minutes grounded
- 30 minutes meditating/breathwork
  - Wim Hof breathing for 5 minutes or so in a comfortable seated position, with your back straight. Repeating a mantra once the breathwork has taken you to a state of euphoria that fits your current goals.
- 10 minutes unusual body movement
  - Planking, lunging, hinging, squatting, isometrically holding, etc.
- 30 minutes of walking
- Drink a glass of mineralized water
  - First thing when you wake up in the morning drink a glass of water with about 1/4 tablespoon of SEA SALT. Himalayan Pink salt or a grey Celtic Sea salt, not your regular iodized table salt.
- Get hot and cold everyday
  - Sweat some and shiver some every day
  - Sweat through external heat exposure or internal heat (exercise).
  - Shiver through cold exposure
- Read 10 pages
  - If it's easier or more convenient for you using an audible book, then go for 30 minutes of listening.

- Reading about health and wellness every day will help to solidify the importance of your wellbeing. The more you learn, the more responsibility you have. Reading and learning will create new neuro pathways in your brain that will help complete your transformation.

You can combine several of these daily _Tranquil Warrior_ tasks to be more efficient if you feel limited on time.

e.g., Barefoot, shorts and a tank top, yoga/ballistic stretching/isometric workout grounded in the grass, in the sun, doing breathwork.

e.g., Barefoot, shorts and a tank, walking barefoot and working on breathwork in the sun after a meal.

e.g., Barefoot, shorts and a tank, walking, in the sun, after a meal, listening to a book

e.g., Barefoot, shorts and a tank, in the sun, reading a book

e.g., It's 100 degrees outside, you do your daily outdoor routine, and you break a good sweat... the _hot_ part of _hot/cold_ is done

e.g., It's -5 degrees and you did your daily sun exposure. The _cold_ routine is done... keep in mind that you should do bite size increments in that low temp, but winter is no excuse to avoid the sun and grounding.

Whatever works best for you, do it different daily, or do it the same. The point is that you just do it. The more time barefoot and connected to the earth the better, you can purchase a grounding sheet or matt that mimics the earths frequency. Sleeping on a grounding sheet will improve sleep quality and healing. My wife and I have been using one for over 3 years now. Mother Earth is truly the best though, there is something special about the direct contact that reduces stress and inflammation in a way that a grounding sheet just can't.

Increasing your daily dose of sun exposure will help, don't burn yourself, be mindful of your skin, don't put sunscreens on unless you must. Utilize clothing and shade if needed. Avoid sunglasses, they impair the way your body perceives the environment, even though you are directly in the sun, your body believes it's in the shade and your skin will be less protected. You can purchase a red-light therapy device to add to your routine as well. You can utilize both near-infra-red and infra-red lights. Walk longer, do more yoga, do more breathwork, lift heavier weights, do more reps, read longer... none of that will hurt you. I don't include SLEEP as a daily task because that's the number one thing you should be doing every day. Sleeping. Greater than 5-6 hours but no more than 9-10 for an adult is generally the most restorative. If you aren't sleeping long enough or good enough *Everything* in your journey is going to be more difficult. Prioritize sleep!

The goal of the daily tasks are simple and direct. You can spend 3 or more hours a day awakening your tranquil warrior, or you can spend just over an hour. It is up to you. Every living organism on this planet must play by the same 24-hour rules. No one has more hours than you, nor do you have more hours than them. It all boils down to how you prioritize the time that you live in. Time is a funny thing; we always talk about time as if we own it. We *have* time, or *don't have* time. But really, time has us. We cannot stop it; all we can do is live in it. We all have a present moment, but we rarely live in it. We live in the past, through our thoughts and emotions and in the future, predicting good and bad outcomes that may never develop. We spend little *time* absolutely in the present. We cannot purchase or acquire any more of it, yet we decide consciously where we *spend* it, and often we waste most of it. The actions that matter most in this awakening are your intention, attention, and perception.

The Mindful Fitness warm-up

-Shake out legs, arms, hands etc. grounding in a strong athletic position

-Tapping – (TWO DEEP BREATHS)

Third eye

Upper cheek bones

Under the collar bones in the corners

Thymus/Heart chakra

Right below rib cage

Upper Thighs – Side thighs

-Crossovers/Crossing

Cross Crawl – Homolateral 20X each leg

Shoulder Crossover-3X each shoulder

Cross Crawl/walk-20X each leg

Flat handed cross body shove (Tai Chi)-20X each side

-Pulling/lymph, blood, energy

Pull Across Eyebrows, forehead, crown and slowly making our way down the neck and onto the traps pulling forward hard, dropping hands heavy and then Restart just above the waistline, moving up the body slowly up the core to the chest, the neck, below chin, chin, mouth, below eyes, eyebrows, Forehead all the way up the head down to the neck and then … rubbing hands together

-Heaven and Earth

Rub your hands together real hard, then shake them off, spread your fingers wide and place them on your thighs, spread your toes out wide and imagine roots coming from your toes and feet grounding you deeply in the earth, Take THREE DEEP BREATHS here...

Reach down and touch the ground, imagining your fingertips connecting deeply with mother earth, take THREE DEEP BREATHS here

Slowly rise, reaching high to the heavens, stretching your fingers and arms and core as far as they will go, take THREE DEEP BREATHS here.

-Zen Swings

With your arms hanging freely to your side, lean forward just a little, begin swaying side to side letting your arms swings out laterally, eventually letting them reach about halfway between your shoulders and hips. Zenfully swing and notice your breath while slightly bending the knees and engaging your obliques.

I normally follow this with three rounds of Wim Hof breathing prior to workouts or to begin my day.

Thank you for reading! Sincerely, Trenton and Kaitlyn Sweet.

BIBLIOGRAPHY

- Trenton Sweet's Life Experiences
- Kaitlyn Sweet's Life Experiences
- A Brief History of Creation, Bill Meslet, James Cleaves
- A Day in the Sex Life of the Hulk Using Gut Microbiome-Sex Connection to Boost Testosterone in Men, Dr Mohamed Kotb
- A new Understanding of the Atom, Professor John T. Sanders
- Almost Human, Lee Berger, John Hawks
- Anatomy of The Spirit, Caroline Myss
- Are We Smart Enough to Know How Smart Animals are?, Frans De Waal
- Astrophysics for People in a Hurry, Neil DeGrasse Tyson
- At the Edge of Uncertainty, Micheal Brooks
- Atlas of a Lost World, Craig Childs
- Atom Land, Jon Butterfield
- Auras, Understand and Feel Them, Marta Tuchowska
- Becoming Supernatural, Dr. Joe Dispenza
- Beyond Training, Ben Greenfield
- Biochemical Individuality, Roger J, Williams PhD
- Bioenergy Healing, Csongor Daniel
- Biology of Belief, Bruce Lipton
- Boundless, Ben Greenfield
- Breaking the Habit of Being Yourself, Dr. Joe Dispenza
- Breath, James Nestor
- Breathing for Warriors, Dr. Belisa Vranich, Brian Sabin
- Burn the Fat, Feed the Muscle, Tom Venuto
- Can't Hurt Me, David Goggins

- CDC.com
- Chakra Healing, Margarita Alcontara
- Chakras, Chakra balancing for busy people, Marta Tuchowska
- Chemistry and our Universe, Ron B. Davis, (Great Courses)
- Civilized to Death, Christopher Ryan
- Clean, James Hamblin
- Deep Nutrition, Catherine Shanahan MD, Luke Shanahan
- Dirt to Soil, Gabe Brown
- Earthing, Matin Zucker, Clinton Ober, Stephen T. Sinatra
- Electric Body, Electric Health, Eileen Day McKusick
- EMF'd, Dr. Joseph Mercola
- Energy Medicine, Donna Eden
- Entangled Minds, Dean Radin PhD
- Evolve your Brain, Dr. Joe Dispenza
- Feeding you Lies, Vani Hari
- Feng Shui Mommy, Bailey Gaddis
- Fit Soul, Ben Greenfield
- Food Babe Kitchen, Vani Hari
- Food of the Gods, Terence McKenna
- Foraging with Kids, Adele Nozedar
- Forest Bathing, Dr. Qing Li
- Gaia, a look at life on Earth, James Lovelock
- GreenMedInfo.com
- Halgamuge MN. Pineal melatonin level disruption. Radiat Prot Dosimetry. 2013 May;154(4):405-16. Doi: 10.1093/rpd/ncs255. Epub 2012 Oct 10. PNID: 23051584.

- Healing Mushrooms, Tero Isokauppila
- Holistic Dental Care, Nadine Artemis
- Holistic Wellness Treatments for Total Welbeing, Marta Tuchowska
- How not to Die, Michael Gregor MD
- How To Train Your Mind, Chris Bailey
- Human Evolution, Charles River Editors
- Kellog, J.H. (1888). Treatment for self-abuse and its effects, in J. H. Kellog, Plain Facts for Old and Young; embracing the natural hystory of organic life (pp. 290-327). I F Segner. https://doi.org/10.1037/12999-023
- Life Force, Tony Robbins, Peter Diamandis, Robert Hariri
- Lifespan, David A. Sinclair
- Living Fully, Mallory Ervin
- Magnolia Table, Joanna Gaines
- Man 2.0 Engineering the Alpha, John Romaniello, Arnold Schwarzenegger
- Mental Combat, Phil Pierce
- Minimize Injury, Maximize Performance, Dr. Tommy John
- Mysteries of the Microscopic World, Bruce Fleury (Great Courses)
- Nourished Beginnings Baby Food, Renee Kohley
- Origins, Frank Rhodes
- Origins, Neil DeGrasse Tyson
- Our Symphony with Animals, Aysha Akhtar MD
- Particle Physics for Non-Physicists, Steven Pollock
- Plant Science, an Introduction to Botany, Catherine Kleier (Great Courses)
- Plant Spirit Medicine, Eliot Cowan

- Quantum Physics, Michael G. Raymer
- Quantum Relativity and the Quantum Revolution, Richard Wolfson
- Quench, Dana Cohen, Gina Bria
- Read it Before you Eat it, Bonnie Taub-Dix
- Regenerate, Sayer Ji
- Reiki and Reiki Meditation, Marta Tuchowska
- Renegade Beauty, Nadine Artemis
- Sacred Earth, Sacred Soul, John Philip Newell
- Sapien, Yuval Noah Harari
- Spiritual Portals, Nor D'Ecclesis
- Superlife, Darin Olien
- The Astrology of you and me, Gary Goldschneider
- The Body Electric, Roberto O. Becker MD, Gary Selder
- The Book of Lymph, Lisa Levitt Gainsley
- The Botany of Desire, Michael Pollan
- The Bulletproof Diet, Dave Asprey
- The Carnivore Code, Paul Saladino MD
- The Case Against Sugar, Gary Taubes
- The Craving Mind, Judson Brewer, John Kabat-Zinn
- The Epigenetic Revolution, Nessa Carrey
- The First Three Minutes, Steven Wienberg
- The Fourth Phase of Water, Gerald Pollack
- The Game of Life and How to Play it, Florence Scovel Shinn
- The Genius Life, Max Lugavere
- The Happiness Hypothesis, Jonathon Haidt
- The Heartbeat of the Trees, Peter Wohlleben
- The History of Sugar, Kelly Fanto Deetz (Great Courses)
- The How not to Die Cookbook, Michael Gregor MD

- The Inflammation Spectrum, Dr. Will Cole, Eve Adamson
- The Intentions Experiment, Lynne McTaggart
- The Longevity Paradox, Steven Gundry MD
- The Lost World of Genesis One, John H. Walton
- The Meateater Fish and Game Cookbook, Steven Rinella
- The Meateater Guide to Wilderness Skills and Survival, Steven Rinella
- The Medicine Bag, Don Jose Ruiz
- The Mind-Gut Connection, Emeran Mayer MD
- The Other Side of History, Daily Life in the Ancient World, Robert Garland (Great Courses)
- The Oxygen Advantage, Patrick McKeown
- The Physics of God, Amit Goswami, Joseph Selbie
- The Quantum Doctor, Deepak Chopra
- The Remarkable Life of the Skin, Monty Lyman
- The Secret Life of Plants, Peter Tompkins and Chrstopher Bird
- The Sleep Solution, Chris Winter MD
- The Story of Human Language, John McWhorter (Great Courses)
- The Theory of Everything, The Question to Explain all Reality, Don Lincoln (Great Courses)
- The Third Chimpanzee, Jared Diamond
- The Three Day Effect, Florence Williams
- The Tibetan Yoga of Breath, Anyen Rinpoche, Allison Choying Zangmo
- The Vegetarian Myth, Lierre Kieth
- The Way of the Iceman, Wim Hof, Koen De Jong
- The Wedge, Scott Carney

- The Whole Brain Child, Daniel J Siegel MD, Tina Payne Bryson PhD
- The Wim Hof Method, Wim Hof
- The Wisdom Codes, Gregg Braden
- The Wisdom of Our Cells, Bruce Lipton
- Think Like a Monk, Jay Shetty
- Transform Your Life, Hypno Sion
- We are all Stardust, Stegan Klein
- WebMd.com
- What do You Care What Other People Think?, Richard P. Feynman, Ralph Leighton
- What Doesn't Kill Us, Scott Carney
- What the Bleep do we Know, William Arntz, Betsy Chase, Mark Vicente
- Who We are and How we Got Here, David Reich
- Whole, Natural Harry
- Why We Get Fat, Gary Taubes
- Wild Magic, Danu Forest
- You are the Guru, Gabby Bernstein
- You are the Placebo, Dr. Joe Dispenza
- You are The Universe, Deepak Chopra MD, Mena C. Kafatos PhD
- Your Spark is Light, Courtney Hunt, MD

CPSIA information can be obtained
at www.ICGtesting.com
Printed in the USA
BVHW050031090223
658189BV00003B/149